Human Heredity and Birth Defects

The Science and Society Series

This series of books, under the general editorship of the Biological Sciences Curriculum Study (BSCS), is for people who have both an interest in biology and a continuing desire to teach themselves. The books are short, highly readable, and nontechnical; each is written by a specialist on a particular, significant aspect of biology. Consistent with a long-standing premise of BSCS, the authors approach their topics as a base for inquiry; they pose questions and help the reader to see the way a scientist arrives at answers or where answers are to be sought. While the books are oriented for the layman primarily, it is hoped that they will also prove useful to high school and college students who wish more background in unfamiliar fields.

There are two major types of books in the series. One of these is directed to the continued and practical problems of society for which biology has both information and a message; topics such as birth control, eugenics and drugs are of personal interest and concern to most individuals. The other cluster of books is devoted to the continuing problems of biology; these topics, such as animal behavior, population biology, and chemical coordination, often relate to societal problems and are of particular concern to biology as a developing discipline. Together, the two clusters give some measure of the totality of modern biology, to which we invite your time and attention.

William V. Mayer
Director, BSCS
Boulder, Colorado

Human Heredity and Birth Defects

E. PETER VOLPE

PEGASUS

A DIVISION OF **Bobbs-Merrill Educational Publishing**
Indianapolis

The Bobbs-Merrill Company, Inc.
4300 West 62nd Street
Indianapolis, Indiana 46268

First Edition
Ninth Printing—1980
Library of Congress Catalog Card Number: 75–124674
ISBN 0–672–63549–6 (pbk.)

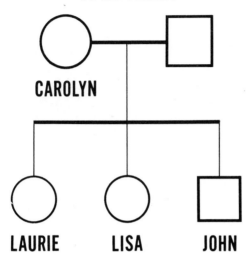

Contents

Editor's Preface

In *Birth Control,* another book in this series, Garrett Hardin puts considerable stress on the concept that every child should be a wanted child. The matter of such planning, however, is complicated by a more serious matter, the one to which Peter Volpe has directed attention in this book. If, as he notes, a deformed child is born every thirty seconds, the deeply personal and poignant concern becomes, "Will my child be normal?"

In a non-technical and sympathetic way, Dr. Volpe has presented the basic issue: the interaction of nature and nurture in the developmental process. Nature, in the form of normal and abnormal genes and of normal and abnormal behavior of chromosomes, interacts with the nurture of the womb and its molecules, diseases, drugs and chemical additives. As he straightforwardly notes, some of these factors are under parental control, others are not. Implicit in discussing the latter is the notion that the uncontrollable could be subject to a different kind of control, that of non-reproduction.

Volpe has discussed the hereditary defects which are generally well-known but poorly understood in terms of cause and control: thalidomide deformities, mongolism, sickle cell anemia. He has also called to attention some defects not generally recognized as inheritable: cystic fibrosis, sexual abnormalities, enzyme-deficiency diseases. His review is comprehensive without being exhaustive, complete without being encyclopedic.

A final epilogue brings the topic into another dimension of personal concern, and one to which society will have to direct its collective concern in the immediate future: the engineering of human heredity by direct interaction with genetic material.

Edward J. Kormondy
Washington, D.C.

Preface

THE EXPECTANT MOTHER is filled with many apprehensive thoughts, but no feeling is more oppressive than the fear of having a deformed baby. A concrete expression of this fear is the question that is almost always asked by the mother immediately after delivery: "Is my baby normal?" Universally, the mother's first look at her newborn infant is an anxious, searching look.

Defects at birth that doom the infant to an early death or a lifetime of illness take an enormous toll of human life and human potential. A deformed child is delivered into the world every thirty seconds. No statistics, however, speak for the psychological trauma suffered by the parents. The birth of a defective child imposes an emotional crisis on the married couple to which adjustment is slow and agonizing. It is difficult to overcome the deep anxieties and unjustified feelings of guilt or shame experienced by the parents. In our affluent society, birth defects still loom as one of man's serious problems.

Interest in birth defects has been heightened in recent years by the "thalidomide" disaster that came to public attention in 1961. A supposedly harmless sleeping pill made of the drug thalidomide, when taken by a pregnant woman, led to a grotesque deformity in her newborn baby. Its arms were absent or reduced to tiny, flipperlike stumps. No longer could it be blandly assumed that the developing infant is tenderly protected in the interior of its mother from drugs in the mother's blood stream, from viruses that infect the mother, or from other environmental disturbances.

The unborn child has no control over the environmental interior furnished it by the mother. Nor, for that matter, does the child have any control over the hereditary potentials transmitted to it by the parents. The child's inherited potentialities, for better or for worse, are established at the time of conception. The unsuspecting child may inherit a defective set of genetic blueprints from its parents, and be cheated of eyes or burdened with extra fingers or toes.

Progress in the treatment of birth deformities has been impressive. Thousands of malformed infants who under more primitive conditions would have died early in life are now saved by the miracles of modern medicine. Less than a year ago, medical researchers were elated by the news that a new special therapy has enabled many infants afflicted with cystic fibrosis to live past childhood into young adult life. Cystic fibrosis is an inherited disorder and one of the major causes of death in children. One child in every thousand is born with this genetic disease. Physicians found particularly encouraging the report that several women patients with cystic fibrosis responded so well to the special treatment that they have now borne children of their own. All these children are normal. If our culture has an ideal, it is the sacredness of human life. But, these normal children born of affected mothers harbor the harmful gene for cystic fibrosis and can pass on the defective gene to their offspring. As these children themselves reach child-bearing age, they will be faced with a choice: to perpetuate the dreaded gene or to avoid pregnancy. Which alternative involves less human suffering?

The choice of alternatives will not be easy. With increasing knowledge, however, the resolution of many such profound problems may become less burdensome. The public is eager for knowledge of new medical breakthroughs on birth defects. Much of the knowledge, however, appears in highly technical scientific papers, not readily accessible to, nor easily understood by, the interested layman. This book has been prepared for the general reader who is not trained in medicine, genetics, or the biological sciences. It has grown out of my experience in teaching students seeking a liberal education—seeking a greater awareness of themselves as persons and of their role in society. It is my hope that accuracy has not been forfeited in the attempt to present a simple, concise account of the present state of research on birth defects and the implications of recent medical advances for the future of man.

E. PETER VOLPE

Tulane University
New Orleans, Louisiana

Acknowledgments

I MUST FIRST THANK Dr. William V. Mayer, Director of the Biological Sciences Curriculum Study, for encouraging me to launch the preparation of this book. The painstaking reading of the entire manuscript was undertaken by Dr. Edward J. Kormondy and Miss Linda Lalor. Mrs. Mary Eastin cheerfully typed the manuscript in its various forms and Mrs. Paula Gebhardt carefully prepared the Index. The drawings are the accomplished work of Mr. Robert Wilson and his art staff of the Biological Sciences Curriculum Study. For photographs, I am indebted to numerous authors and publishers for their generosity and cooperation. Specific credit for individual photographs has been given in the caption under each picture. My greatest debt is to my wife for help and encouragement in more ways than I can enumerate.

E. P. V.

Chapter 1

Seeds of Life

CONGENITAL DEFECTS, or deformities present at birth, have shocked and fascinated people since the dawn of history. Primitive hunters of the Stone Age sketched vivid pictures of grotesque human forms on the walls of caves. Ancient tribesmen of the Mesopotamian and Nile valleys engraved double-headed creatures on baked clay tablets. Dwarfed infants were depicted in Egyptian paintings 5,000 years old.

Superstition and witchcraft shrouded early man's desire to understand strange abnormalities. Grossly distorted infants were graphically described as "monsters," from the Latin word *monstrum*, meaning a sinister omen or marvel. Bizarre one-eyed or two-headed babies (FIG. 1-1) were solemnly regarded as the vengeful acts of an angry deity. The malformed babies, possessed of evil spirits, were either left to perish by exposure in the mountains or cast into the rivers and seas. Infanticide, or the killing of a sickly infant, was a common and socially approved practice. This ritualistic practice, like all rituals, was devised to overcome man's feelings of powerlessness and helplessness in matters over which he recognized he had no direct control or influence.

In the heroic Greek age, it was fashionable to attribute the birth of monsters to women having been impregnated by lower forms of animals. This was in keeping with the old Hindu idea that a child was molded out of the mother's menstrual blood under the organizing influence of the semen. Obviously the semen of a wild animal could only distort the menstrual fluid into odd shapes. Aristotle (384–322 B.C.), the great philosopher and naturalist, did not deny that a human and a brute form could mate, but argued unconvincingly that offspring would not be generated because of different lengths of the child-carrying (gestation) period.

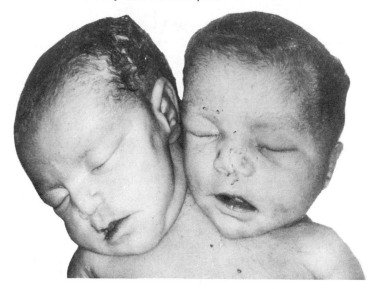

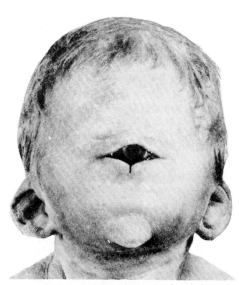

FIG. 1-1 GROTESQUE CONGENITAL DEFORMITIES: two-headed newborn infant *(top)* and cyclopean, or one-eyed, infant *(bottom)*. *(Top,* Courtesy of Dr. Norman Woody, Tulane University School of Medicine; *Bottom,* from E. L. Potter, *Pathology of the Fetus and the Infant,* Year Book Medical Publishers, ©1961 used by permission.)

Fanciful stories of instances of human intercourse with lower animals—such as goats and snakes—remained in vogue into medieval times. Incredible tales continued to be told about how serpents sprung from women's hair or how half-human offspring came from women that had been abducted by apes. Many semi-human creatures were invented or imagined. According to one legend, there was born in 1493, as the result of intercourse between a woman and a dog, a creature resembling in its upper extremities its mother, while its lower extremities were the exact counterpart of its canine father (FIG. 1-2).

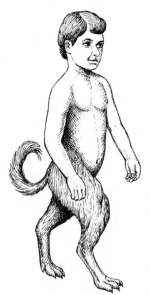

FIG. 1-2 BOY-DOG, the fanciful offspring of a woman who had been impregnated by a dog, based on a legend attributed to the noted fifteenth-century surgeon Ambroise Paré. Stories of human beings having intercourse with animals are recorded innumerable times in medieval medical history.

Throughout the dark Middle Ages, from about the years 900 to 1500, belief and dependence on magic and witchcraft still dominated man's thoughts and behavior. Harsh treatment was prescribed for deformed infants as well as for their mothers. Women were burned at the stake for the alleged crime of giving birth to a malformed child. Certain deformed individuals were spared, but for the wrong reasons. Dwarfs, looked upon as droll, were often kept as court jesters by the nobility.

In the 17th century, the discovery of wriggly sperm in the semen aroused new speculations. Human sperm were seen for the first time in 1677 by the Dutchman Anton van Leeuwenhoek (1632–1723), a merchant who polished lenses as a hobby and assiduously made more than 200 simple microscopes. Leeuwenhoek and his colleagues were victimized by imperfect lenses and a fertile imagination. Many learned men of the day imagined that the sperm contained a tiny replica of a human individual. The function of a woman's womb was simply to protect and nourish the preformed diminutive human until it unfolded into the adult form. Enthusiasts of the idea actually portrayed the imaginary human figure (FIG. 1–3) and even invented a name for it: "homunculus," or "little man." Other

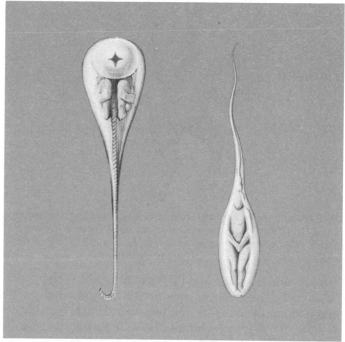

FIG. 1–3 SPECULATIVE DRAWINGS from the eighteenth century which show the human sperm harboring a fully formed, diminutive being.

scientists contended that the preformed human being resided rather in the egg (or ovum) and that the sperm served solely to stimulate the little individual to grow. During the 18th century the sharp differences of opinion over the location of the preformed child degenerated into an intellectual muddle.

It was not until the first half of the 19th century that the absurd "little man," or "homunculus," was finally laid to rest by the realization that both the sperm and egg are necessary for the initiation of development. In the 1830's, two German biologists, Theodor Schwann (1810–1882) and Matthias Schleiden (1804–1881), reached the major conclusion that all living things, whether a moth, an oak tree, or man, are composed of structural units known as cells. The new individual begins life as a single cell, the fertilized egg, which itself is formed by the fusion of two cells: the sperm and the egg. The union of these two gametes, as they are often called, sets in motion a chain of events that gives rise to a new being. There is no preformed visible pattern in the fertilized egg. There is no hint of the form that is eventually to emerge.

It is remarkable that within the small compass of the fertilized human egg, about 0.14 millimeter (1/175 inch) in diameter and weighing four millionths of a gram (0.000004 gram), there reside the potentialities of development into a complete human being. The fertilized egg (or zygote) divides into two, the two into four, the four into eight, and so on until the number of cells has multiplied into billions. The cells become specialized and congregate into tissues—such as muscle and nerve—and, in turn, the tissues interact to form a variety of organs—such as heart and liver. The organs intermesh to produce the characteristic form of the body. At the time of birth, the human fetus has 200 billion cells and weighs about 3,000 million times as much as the fertilized egg. The average infant at term weighs 3,200 grams (7 pounds), males being roughly 100 grams (3 ounces) heavier than females.

Development of an individual is truly a complicated affair involving the delicate integration of many processes. The birth of an occasional infant with a defective heart or extra fingers excites surprise and wonder. The primary wonder, however, is that the intricate developmental processes should proceed in an orderly normal fashion in the great majority of cases. Medical scientists still marvel that deformities are not the rule rather than the exception.

The Human Egg

THE MOST EXTRAORDINARY bits of living matter are the sperm and egg cells. The tadpole-shaped human sperm is too minute to be seen without the aid of a high-powered microscope. In fact, it is the smallest cell in the human body, with a total length of 1/500 of an inch. The spherical human egg is barely visible to the unaided eye; it is smaller than the dot of a fine pencil and would be recognized only by a trained observer. Nobel Laureate Hermann J. Muller (1890–1967) once remarked that two billion sperm closely packed together would make no larger bulk than half of an ordinary aspirin tablet. A comparable number of eggs could be comfortably placed in a teaspoon. Yet these two tiny blobs of protoplasm comprise the sole perpetuators of life.

Under the microscope the human egg is seen as a globule of protoplasm (more specifically, cytoplasm) surrounded by a

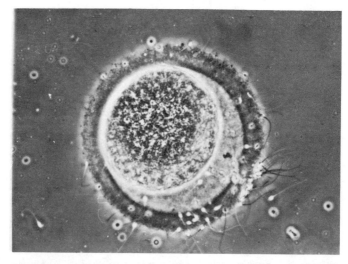

FIG. 1–4 HUMAN EGG, shown here 4,000 times actual size, is surrounded by sperm in the Fallopian tube. (Courtesy of Dr. Landrum B. Shettles, College of Physicians and Surgeons, Columbia University.)

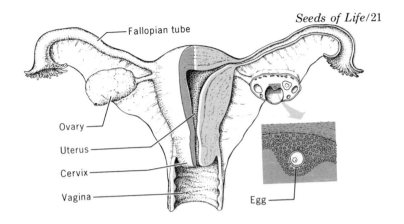

FIG. 1-5 HUMAN OVARY, with enlarged view of egg, and its associated genital tract.

thick translucent envelope (FIG. 1-4). By special techniques the egg can be shown to contain a spherical body, the nucleus, which plays a prominent role in heredity. Scattered fat droplets (yolk) impart a granular appearance to the egg. Compared to a hen's egg, the amount of yolk in the human egg is exceedingly meager. In humans, the mother replaces yolk as the source of nutrition for the embryo.

Women contain many more eggs than they need in their reproductive life. The paired, almond-shaped ovaries (FIG. 1-5) harbor somewhere between 100,000 and 600,000 eggs, of which about 400 are released during a woman's fertile years. Ovulation, the liberation of the egg from the ovary, occurs once in every 28-day cycle of the mature woman. An egg is released typically on the 13th-14th day after the beginning of the preceding menstrual period. There are unpredictable variations in the onset of ovulation. The discharge of the egg has been reported to occur as early as the sixth day (counting from the first day of the preceding menstruation) and as late as the 23rd day.

In contrast to most other forms of animal life, sexual receptivity in the human female is not related to ovulation. Most mammals mate only during a restricted season or period. The female dog, for example, will copulate only when she ovulates ("comes into heat"), once every six or seven months, and offspring are almost always assured. The human female is not confined to receiving the male only during the period of ovulation. Ignoring cultural mores, she can be receptive to the male throughout her 28-day cycle.

Typically only one egg escapes at ovulation, either from one ovary or the other. Save for a possible slight abdominal pain, most women are unaware that they have ovulated. The liberated egg is swept into one of the Fallopian tubes, the narrow ducts which extend from the ovaries to the pear-shaped uterus, or womb. Fertilization of the egg normally occurs in the upper reaches of the Fallopian tube. The egg is capable of being fertilized for only a few hours, as judged by the brief period of competence of other mammalian eggs. The eggs of guinea pigs are known to degenerate as early as eight hours after ovulation, whereas rabbit eggs do not survive for more than six hours. Thus, if conception is to occur in the human, fertilization must take place within 12 to 24 hours of ovulation.

If the egg has been fertilized, it burrows its way into the thick, spongy wall of the uterus. The uterus, rich in blood vessels, is fully prepared at this time to nourish a young embryo. If conception has not taken place, the egg deteriorates and the lining of the uterus is sloughed off in menstruation. One scho-

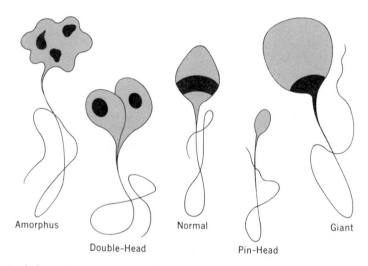

Amorphus

Double-Head

Normal

Pin-Head

Giant

FIG. 1–6 NORMAL AND ABNORMAL human sperm cells. When the percentage of abnormal types in the male semen exceeds 25 percent, the male is sterile.

larly wit has described the sloughing and hemorrhaging of the uterine lining as the "protest of a disappointed uterus."

The duration of the menstrual flow is variable, the usual length of time being four to six days. There is no semblance of scientific truth to the early concept that the menstrual flow contains a toxic substance. This view is traceable to the writings of the early Greeks and Romans. In those times and as late as the 16th century, menstruating women were shunned, obliged to seclude themselves, and forbidden to touch anything. Menstrual blood was believed to be so potent that the mere touch of a menstruating woman would render all kinds of life sterile. Pliny (A.D. 23–79), the erudite Roman naturalist, said that "seeds which are touched (by a menstruating woman) become sterile, grass withers away, garden plants are parched up, and the fruit will fall from the tree beneath which she sits." No such views are held (or tolerated) today.

The Human Sperm

THE HUMAN SPERM CELL is admirably constructed for the herculean task of traveling to and penetrating the egg. The highly motile sperm bear little resemblance to the ordinary or typical cell (FIG. 1–6). In fact, they were first described as animalcules, or "little animals." The sperm cell has an oval "head," within which is the nucleus; a "neck," which is the source of energy for the sperm's vigorous movements; and a long, thin tail which lashes from side to side. Sperm are produced in small, convoluted tubules (seminiferous tubules) inside each of the two testes. The commonly used term "testicle" is an exact synonym of "testis," but the latter is almost invariably preferred in scientific writing. The word testicle was once applied as well to the ovary of the female. Prior to the introduction of the term "ovary" in 1672 by the Dutch scientist Reinier de Graaf (1641–1673), the expression "female testicle" was used in reference to the female organ.

The sperm mature and become motile in a maze of highly coiled tubules located on one side of each testis. Sperm ultimately reach the exterior through a narrow tube (the urethra), which functions also to convey urine. In their passage through various ducts, the sperm are mixed with the viscid secretions of special glands, including the prostate. This whitish mixture constitutes the semen (from the Latin root of *serere,* "to sow").

The sperm are actively motile in the fluid of the female genital tract where they swim against the current, tadpole fashion, at an estimated speed of one-tenth of an inch a minute. They have a limited life span in the female genital tract. Their capacity for swimming may last up to three or four days, but their fertilizing capability is probably lost within 24 hours. The fertilizing span of sperm in most mammals is typically short, as brief as six hours in the mouse. A notable exception is the bat, whose sperm, deposited in the fall, can actually winter over in the female tract until eggs are ovulated in the spring.

Sperm are produced in the testes in unbelievable quantity. A single ejaculate may contain as many as 350 million sperm. A minimum of 80 million motile sperm per ejaculate is considered necessary for fertility. Not all sperm cells produced are morphologically alike; indeed, ejaculates typically contain a variety of sperm types, of which only one kind is normal (FIG. 1–6). When the percentage of abnormal types in an ejaculate is in excess of 25 percent, the male is sterile. As many as four out of every 10 infertile marriages may be due primarily to an inadequate sperm count and poor sperm morphology.

Although innumerable sperm are produced, comparatively few—as few as three or four—actually reach the site of fertilization in the Fallopian tubes. Most meet death or entrapment as they pass from the vagina through the uterus and into the Fallopian tubes. Only one of the vast numbers of sperm successfully penetrates the egg. The head of the sperm, containing the nucleus, enters the egg; the tail, its mission accomplished, becomes detached and disintegrates. The nucleus of the sperm then unites with the nucleus of the egg. At that moment, the fertilization process is completed.

The Genetic Blueprints

HIPPOCRATES, the learned Greek physician of the fifth century B.C., recognized that both the mother and father make a contribution to their offspring. He erred, however, in asserting that the male and female furnish unequal amounts of "semen," and that the child will most resemble the parent who contributed the most semen. Although the egg is many times greater in volume than the sperm, the two have equal potentialities as far as inheritance is concerned. The blueprints for traits are carried in the nucleus of each gamete. The genetic characteristics of the future child are established at the time the sperm nucleus unites with the egg nucleus.

Knowledge of the internal organization of the nucleus came slowly to science. Its advance depended primarily on the perfection of the microscope and the development of techniques to stain the cell with various dyes. The most significant visible components of the nucleus are threadlike strands, termed chromosomes, so named because of their affinity for certain dyes (Greek, "colored bodies"). Every form of life has a definite and characteristic number of chromosomes. The fruit fly has 8 in every body cell, the frog has 26, and man has 46. The chromosomes occur in pairs in each body cell; hence, man has 23 pairs. One member of each pair comes from the mother and the other from the father. Stated another way, the gametes each have only half the number of chromosomes of the

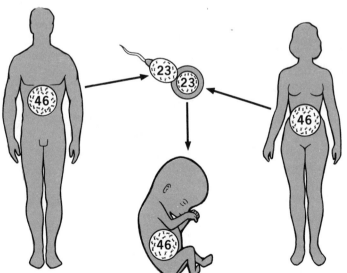

FIG. 1–7 THE NEWBORN contains 46 chromosomes, having received 23 chromosomes from the mother and 23 from the father.

parents. Fertilization restores the original number and the paired condition (FIG. 1-7). The 46 chromosomes of the fertilized egg are passed on to all the cells during development, so that all cells of the adult have the same number.

It is now well documented that the actual material responsible for the determination of traits are submicroscopic molecules, the genes, arranged in a linear sequence in the chromosomes. The gene responsible for a particular trait has a specific position, or "locus," in the chromosome. Each chromosome contains several hundred genes. A conservative estimate would place the total number of genes in man at 20,000. Like the chromosomes, the genes occur in pairs. The fertilized egg carries two representatives of each kind of gene, one from each parent. This fact forms one of the cornerstones in the foundation of the science of genetics, as will be seen in more detail later.

For the moment, the important consideration is that genes are the controllers of development. During the division of the fertilized egg cell into many daughter cells, the genes regularly produce copies of themselves with each cell division. As a result, each of the millions of cells of the developing embryo carries faithful copies of the genes of the fertilized egg. Unfortunately, errors in copying do occasionally occur, resulting in defective genes and the threat of a deformed baby.

Genes determine the infinite detail of bodily structure. It should be understood that genes have no eyes, no legs, nor brains. Genes are essentially minute chemical factories. What genes direct are chemical processes which result ultimately in the emergence of bodily structures. Genes, thus, prescribe only a potentiality for a trait. The environment of the developing embryo determines how well the genetic potentiality is realized. As soon as the fertilized egg begins to divide and grow, it is subjected to an environment furnished by the mother. *The environment in the womb can foster—or cripple—the inherited tendencies of the developing embryo.*

Chapter 2

Embryonic and Fetal Development

LIFE BEGINS WHEN a sperm unites with the egg in the Fallopian tube. It takes the fertilized egg nearly a week to find its way into the wall of the uterus. Three or four days are spent journeying through the Fallopian tube, during which time the egg has divided several times. The embryo, no longer an egg but a spherical cluster of cells, floats about in the cavity of the uterus for another three or four days before sinking into the wall. Not all of the fertilized eggs survive the tumultuous first week. Current evidence indicates that as many as 50 percent of the fertilized eggs fail to implant properly.

The embryo is wholly dependent for its survival and growth on the mother. Once lodged in the uterine wall, the embryo quickly establishes an intimate relation with the mother's blood stream. Many of the embryonic cells migrate out, far beyond the region of the embryo itself, to form what are known as extraembryonic membranes. These, as the name implies, are not incorporated in the body of the embryo and are cast off at the time of birth.

One important extraembryonic membrane is the amnion, a layer of cells which envelops the growing embryo and becomes filled with a watery fluid. The fluid-filled amnionic sac serves as a cushion which protects the embryo from mechanical injury and, at the same time, allows it freedom of motion. The amnionic sac, or "bag," typically ruptures during birth, liberating the "waters." Very rarely the head of the child is born with the unbroken amnion still surrounding it like a veil, a condition which has long been superstitiously considered an omen of good luck.

Another vital extraembryonic membrane is the chorion, which fuses with the lining of the uterus to form the placenta or "afterbirth." Fingerlike projections of the chorion, known as chorionic villi, penetrate deeply into the uterine wall and come to lie in the maternal blood spaces. The chorionic villi form an extensive treelike system (FIG. 2–1). Blood vessels of the embryo protrude into the chorionic villi, thereby bringing the embryonic blood close to the mother's blood. But at no time during pregnancy is there an intermingling of the blood of mother and child. To the placenta, the mother's blood stream carries nutritive food and oxygen, while conversely the embryo's vessels convey carbon dioxide and nitrogenous waste products of metabolism. The mother disposes of her child's wastes through her lungs and kidneys. The placenta also serves as a formidable barrier against harmful substances that may be present in the mother's blood stream. Unfortunately, as we will see later, the placenta may not hold back all noxious substances.

The embryo does not have limitless space in which to grow. At first straight, the embryo becomes markedly bent or curled, head to tail. The formation of the embryonic body as seen externally is illustrated in FIGURE 2–2. The four-week-old embryo bears no resemblance to a human being. The head is vaguely

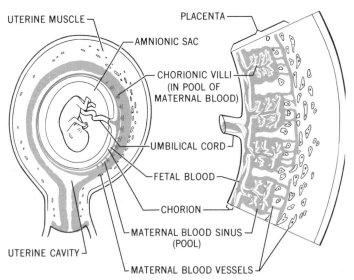

FIG. 2–1 PART OF THE HUMAN PLACENTA, revealing that the blood of the fetus and the blood of the mother circulate independently in totally separate channels.

defined, but it bears a primitive two-lobed brain. A prominent bulge in the trunk region signifies the early beginnings of the heart. The simple-looped heart is functional, pumping blood

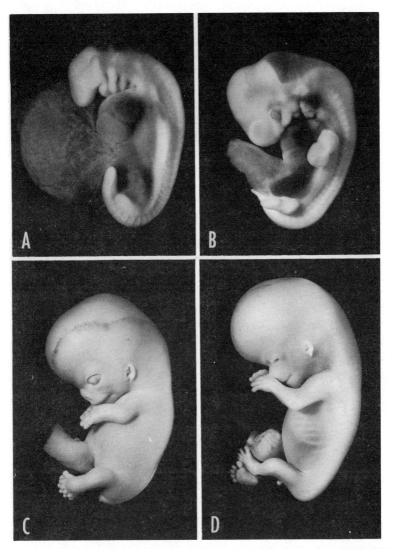

FIG. 2–2 HUMAN EMBRYO at various stages of development: fourth week (A), fifth week (B), sixth week (C), and eighth week (D). (Courtesy of the Carnegie Institution of Washington, Baltimore, Maryland.)

through vessels within the embryo and through special vessels, the umbilical arteries, to the placenta. Vague, rounded elevations on the surface of the head foreshadow the development of the eyes. Although functionless, oral and anal openings arise at this time.

A characteristic feature of the four-week-old embryo (FIG. 2-2*A*) is the presence of an alternating series of ridges and furrows on the sides of the head, known as branchial arches and branchial grooves. The branchial grooves correspond to the gill slits of fishes. However, the grooves in humans are not normally perforated nor do they ever function in respiration. The branchial arches of the human embryo contribute ultimately to several important structures in the facial region; the first arch, for example, is involved in the formation of the upper and lower jaws.

The rudiments of the arms and legs appear about the middle of the fifth week. They arise as two pairs of flattened elevations, known as limb buds (FIG. 2-2*B*). Behind the hind limb bud may be seen a small tail rudiment, which does not ever grow into a full-fledged tail. The head is now appreciably larger than the trunk; the brain has become the most prominent feature of the embryo.

In the sixth week, the head is disproportionately large, the abdomen bulges because of the great size of the liver, and digits are evident in the paddle-shaped hands and feet (FIG. 2-2*C*). The hands are always a little ahead of the feet in their development. This is an expression of the general rule that anterior structures develop more rapidly than posterior structures. Rapid growth and development has occurred in the facial region. The eyes and external ears are well defined, the upper lip has formed, and the nose has definition. In the eighth week (FIG. 2-2*D*), the head is recognizably human: eyes, ears, nose, and mouth are relatively well formed. The tail of earlier stages has regressed.

By the end of the eighth week, all the organs of the body are well established. The embryo is remarkably complex, even though it is only three-fourths of an inch long. The developing individual has a form that is unmistakably human, and thenceforth until birth, seven months later, is known as a fetus. The fetal period is one primarily of growth and refinement of struc-

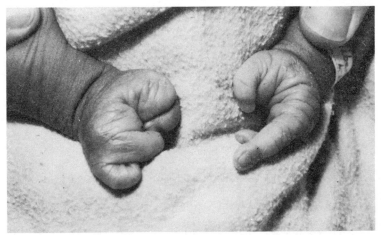

FIG. 2–3 PINCER-LIKE DEFORMITY of a newborn infant's hands, once naïvely attributed to terrifying mental impressions of the mother during pregnancy. Modern knowledge rules out any possibility that the expectant mother can adversely influence her child's development by her imaginative thoughts or fantasies. (Courtesy of Dr. Norman Woody, Tulane University School of Medicine.)

tures formed during the first eight weeks. The total gestation period averages 267 days, with a range of 250 to 310 days.

It bears emphasizing that the child is almost completely formed by the time it completes its eighth week of development. This fact alone is sufficient to reveal the absurdity of the popular and long-persisting belief in maternal impressions or "old wives' tales." A five-month fetus is no more likely to develop a strawberry-shaped birthmark from a mother's yearning for strawberries than is the mother herself. Nor can the infant develop a clawlike deformity of the hands (FIG. 2–3) because the mother was frightened in her sixth month of pregnancy by a packet of live lobsters.

Incidence of Congenital Malformations

HOSPITAL RECORDS in widely scattered parts of the world reveal that approximately one percent of all infants born alive suffer serious disorders ranging from harelip to an extreme condition in which the bony braincase and brain are absent (anencephaly). In other words, one baby in 100 is born with a defect so serious that the infant either dies or is severely handicapped. In the United States alone, 250,000 infants are delivered each year with significant birth defects.

The kinds of major deformities that are common in newly born infants are listed in FIGURE 2–4. More than one-third of

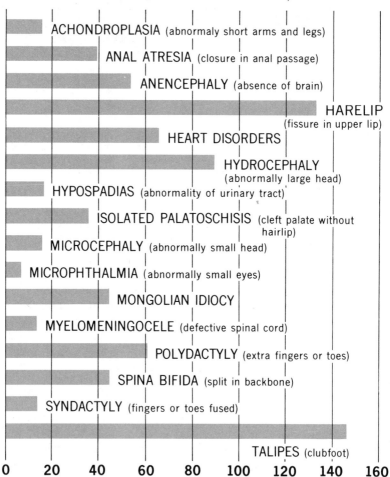

NUMBER OF DEFORMED INFANTS PER 100,000 BIRTHS

ACHONDROPLASIA (abnormaly short arms and legs)

ANAL ATRESIA (closure in anal passage)

ANENCEPHALY (absence of brain)

HARELIP
(fissure in upper lip)

HEART DISORDERS

HYDROCEPHALY
(abnormally large head)

HYPOSPADIAS (abnormality of urinary tract)

ISOLATED PALATOSCHISIS (cleft palate without hairlip)

MICROCEPHALY (abnormally small head)

MICROPHTHALMIA (abnormally small eyes)

MONGOLIAN IDIOCY

MYELOMENINGOCELE (defective spinal cord)

POLYDACTYLY (extra fingers or toes)

SPINA BIFIDA (split in backbone)

SYNDACTYLY (fingers or toes fused)

TALIPES (clubfoot)

0   20   40   60   80   100   120   140   160

FIG. 2–4 MAJOR CONGENITAL DEFORMITIES based on a survey of 44,109 births at University Hospitals in Lund, Sweden. (Compiled by Dr. J. A. Book, Director of the State Institute for Human Genetics in Uppsala, Sweden.)

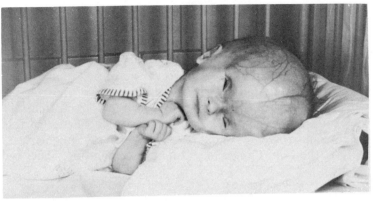

FIG. 2–5 HYDROCEPHALY, a birth defect characterized by abnormal accumulation of fluid in the brain cavities, accompanied by enlargement of the head, deterioration of the brain, and convulsions. (Courtesy of Dr. Norman Woody, Tulane University School of Medicine.)

the malformed babies exhibit defects of the brain and spinal cord. One of the more frequent malformations is hydrocephaly, a condition in which the head is greatly enlarged because of excess fluid in the brain cavities (FIG. 2–5). Other common defects are harelip (with or without cleft palate), polydactyly (extra digits on the hands or feet), and clubfoot (FIG. 2–6). Infants with congenital defects are born prematurely about three times as often as normal infants.

The above statistics are based on live births, and give no indication of the number of deformed embryos lost through spontaneous abortions early in pregnancy. Recent estimates indicate that one in 10 pregnancies terminate in miscarriage. Moreover, many anomalies are not noticeable at birth. Some manifest themselves during the first year after birth; others appear only after many years. An obstruction of the intestinal tract, known as infantile hypertrophic pyloric stenosis, develops in the neonatal period, between the third and seventh week after birth. The inherited degenerative disease of the nervous system, known as Huntington's chorea, first reveals itself in persons in their late thirties. When we group together the figures reported for fetal mortality (stillbirths and abortions), the malformations present in infants at birth, and the deformities that do not become manifest until later life, the total or overall percentage of major deformities in humans is about 5 percent, or one in 20!

The incidence of malformations varies widely in different ethnic groups and in different parts of the world. Spina bifida, in which the spine fails to close over and a gap is left in the spinal column, occurs at least twice as often in Caucasians as in Negroes and twelve times as often as in Japanese. On the other hand, polydactyly is seven times more frequent in Negroes than in Caucasians. Infantile amaurotic idiocy is

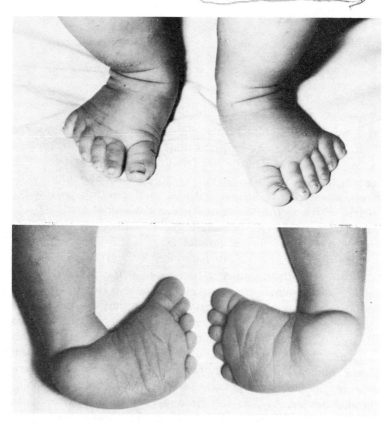

FIG. 2-6 CONGENITAL MALFORMATIONS OF THE FOOT: polydactyly (*top*), characterized by an additional toe, and talipes (*bottom*), in which the foot is twisted out of shape (clubfoot). (Courtesy of Dr. Norman Woody, Tulane University School of Medicine.)

almost confined to Jewish communities in Europe, and harelip and cleft palate occur more frequently in Japan than in any other country. The reasons for these irregularly distributed incidences are still obscure.

The age of the pregnant mother has a decided bearing on the occurrence of certain malformations. The incidence of hydrocephaly and mongolism increases markedly with advancing age. Women above 35 years of age are eight times more apt to have a mongoloid child than women under 25. In other congenital deformities, such as cleft palate and spina bifida, there is no evidence of association with the age of the mother.

The malformation rate is higher among males than females. Some malformations occur predominately in females. Anencephaly (absence of the brain), congenital dislocation of the hips, and spina bifida are far more common in female infants than in male infants, whereas males are more often afflicted with clubfoot and pyloric stenosis. The influence of sex is not fully understood. An excess of females with anencephaly may mean either that females are more vulnerable or that afflicted males are less likely to reach term.

Causes of Congenital Malformations

A TRAIT DOES NOT suddenly emerge, but arises after an orderly sequence of developmental processes or steps. Each step is controlled by one or more genes. The formation of the upper lip, for example, involves many genes and many precisely interwoven reactions. Each gene is only one link in the development of the upper lip. Whether a normal upper lip develops depends on at least two circumstances. The genes may be normal, but some infectious or toxic agent in the maternal environment may disrupt the delicate interlocked embryonic processes. The result may be an anomaly of the upper lip, such as that seen in infants with harelip. On the other hand, the uterine environment may be favorable, but one or more of the genes may be defective. An abnormal gene may retard or prevent some key reaction at a critical point in development. The end result may be the same: a malformation of the upper lip.

The development of an organ or part may be compared to the assemblage of a car in a factory. The assembly line must move with a definite speed, as must the developmental processes. At precise intervals a particular piece must be attached at the proper site. If one piece is left out at a given time, all subsequent operations are hindered and the final outcome is a faulty vehicle or no car at all. Similarly, a defective gene or a noxious environmental agent may either utterly destroy the whole fabric of development or alter the synchronized processes to the extent of producing a malformed bodily part.

A genetically determined malformation is foreordained at the time of fertilization. An environmentally determined anomaly originates from injury to the embryo at a vulnerable stage in its development. It is often quite difficult to ascertain which of the two factors—inheritance of defective genes or adverse effects of external influences—has played the major role in the appearance of the deformity. Unfavorable environmental factors may produce malformations that are similar to those resulting from a defective gene. Moreover, an abnormal gene does not invariably produce the detrimental effect that might have been expected. Under certain environmental conditions, the defective gene may not express itself or cause only a minor, scarcely noticeable, abnormality. One aspect is certain: *the vast majority of deformities originate at an early stage of embryonic development, even before the mother may suspect that she is pregnant. The crucial period of development precedes the eighth week of pregnancy, before any visible sign of the trait itself.*

Chapter 3

Environmentally Determined Abnormalities

SCIENTISTS WORKING WITH experimental animals in the laboratory have known for a long time that developmental abnormalities can arise by changing the environment of the egg or embryo. More than a century ago, in 1832, the French biologist Étienne Geoffroy Saint-Hilaire (1772–1844) sealed with varnish the air pores in the shell of a hen's egg, and observed that the embryo, deprived of its oxygen supply, became deformed. In 1892, the German scientist Hans Driesch (1867–1941) created double-headed embryos by placing the eggs of sea urchins in uncommonly warm water. At the turn of the century, the American biologist Charles R. Stockard (1879–1939) produced the cyclopean (one-eyed) anomaly in fish by culturing the embryos in sea water containing excessive amounts of salt (FIG. 3–1). In the last two decades investigators have directed their efforts to inducing embryonic defects in mammals, particularly in guinea pigs, mice, and rats. Pregnant mice which had been treated with drugs, hormones, or

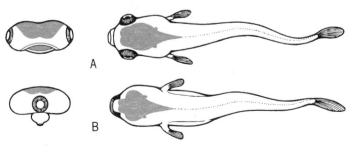

FIG. 3–1 NORMAL (A) AND ABNORMAL (B) DEVELOPMENT of the eye of the Atlantic Coast minnow. The cyclopean (one-eyed) deformity results when the embryo develops in sea water containing an excess amount of a particular salt (magnesium chloride). (Based on studies in 1909 by Dr. C. R. Stockard.)

chemical compounds, or had been exposed to X rays or ultrasonic sound, regularly delivered grossly misshapen offspring. The number of chemical and physical agents, collectively called "teratogens," that are capable of causing malformations of the fetuses in experimental animals has become bewilderingly large.

As late as 1960, most obstetricians were either cautious or blandly complacent about directly extending observations on lower animals to the human. The prevailing feeling was that the human embryo, sheltered in the interior of its mother, appeared to be well protected from all the drastic environmental disturbances to which investigators subjected the embryos of lower forms. Only in recent years has it become distressingly clear that the human embryo can be injured by agents that are tolerated by, or even innocuous to, the mother. This was dramatically revealed in 1961 when medical researchers shockingly discovered that a supposedly harmless sleeping pill made of the drug thalidomide, when taken by a pregnant woman, could lead to a grotesque deformity in the newborn—the baby is cheated of its arms or legs.

The Crippling Drug, Thalidomide

In 1957 a pharmaceutical firm in Stolberg, Germany, marketed a new sleeping pill, made of the drug thalidomide, guaranteed to provide a restful night's sleep without hangover. The manufacture of the pill was licensed in other countries, and

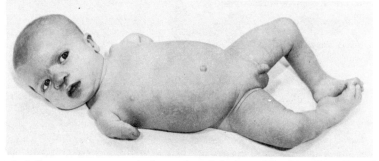

FIG. 3-2 ARMLESS DEFORMITY in the newborn infant, resulting from the action of thalidomide, a sedative taken by his mother in her second month of pregnancy. (Courtesy of Dr. W. Lenz, University of Münster, Germany.)

the pill became available in more than 40 countries over a period of four years. The sleep-inducing drug was advertised as absolutely harmless even for pregnant women. But no evidence of its safety existed, and its toxic effects were soon to become apparent.

In 1959 there occurred sporadic, seemingly unrelated, cases of a peculiar deformity in newborn babies. The babies' arms were absent or reduced to tiny, flipperlike stumps (FIG. 3–2). In some infants the legs were similarly affected; in most instances the deformity of the legs was less severe. In very harsh cases, both arms and legs were missing. The external ear was sometimes malformed and obstructive lesions of the intestine were common. Mentality was normal in the vast majority of the afflicted infants. This rare condition is phocomelia, literally "seal limbs," from the Greek words *phokos* meaning "seal" and *melos* meaning "extremities."

By 1961 the incidence of phocomelia rose sharply in West Germany. In one pediatric clinic alone, in Hamburg, 154 cases were reported in a short span of months in 1961. Obstetricians sought frantically for a cause. By the end of 1961, Dr. Widukind Lenz, Director of the University Clinic for Children in Hamburg, tracked down thalidomide as the one common factor in the catastrophic outbreak of phocomelia. All mothers of the deformed babies had taken thalidomide in the early stages of pregnancy, during the critical period in development when the infant's arms and legs are formed.

At the 1961 Pediatric Meeting at Dusseldorf, Dr. Lenz reported his suspicion that thalidomide was the teratogenic agent. In his speech Dr. Lenz did not name the drug, but it became quickly known among German physicians that thalidomide was the drug under suspicion. Almost simultaneously, and independently, the Australian pediatrician W. G. McBride gave the alarm of the crippling effects of thalidomide from the other side of the world. In November 1961 the drug was withdrawn from the market in Germany. The United States was largely spared the thalidomide disaster by the astute scientific sense of Dr. Frances O. Kelsey of the U.S. Food and Drug Administration. She had wisely blocked general distribution of the drug. Despite her efforts American women did obtain the drug from European sources. Although relatively rare in the

United States, more than 5,000 thalidomide babies were born in West Germany and at least 1,000 in other countries. The deformity was reported from widely different parts of the world—Australia, Scotland, England, Canada, Belgium, Switzerland, Lebanon, Israel, and Peru. Some of the thalidomide babies died, some were put to death, and most have now learned to manage the business of living with the aid of artificial limbs and special training.

There is scarcely any doubt that the tissues of the embryo, at certain stages in differentiation, are extremely sensitive to thalidomide. Dr. Lenz has made a careful study of the types of defects in relation to the time of intake of the drug. The sensitive period of the embryo to thalidomide falls between the 34th and 50th days after the last menstrual period (approximately the third to fourth week of embryonic life). Relatively early intake, between the 34th and 38th days, is associated primarily with gross abnormalities of the ears. Serious damage to the arms resulted when the drug had been taken between the 39th and 44th days. In most cases of deformities of the long bones of the legs thalidomide had been taken between the 44th and 48th days. Disturbances of the intestinal tract and heart defects were common when mothers had used the drug between the 40th and 45th days.

Many of the women had taken thalidomide during the period when they were unaware that they were pregnant. Only one or two tablets (a single dose of 100 milligrams!) has been shown to be sufficient to cause phocomelia. It would appear sensible to adhere to an old adage in medicine: no barbiturates, opiates, sedatives, or hypnotics should be prescribed for, or taken by, mothers-to-be.

Tragedy of German Measles

GERMAN MEASLES—or in medical parlance, "rubella"—is a relatively mild disease caused by a virus. The lymph glands behind the ears swell, rose-pink rashes develop, and a slight fever occurs. Although German measles is a disease of children, it can be contracted by adults. Some adults become infected without displaying any symptoms of the disease. This, we shall see, is particularly unfortunate for mothers in the child-bearing age.

In 1940, Australia was hit by a widespread epidemic of rubella. A year after the outbreak, the Australian ophthalmologist Norman McAlister Gregg drew attention to an alarming number of cases of congenital cataract in newborn infants. The lens of the infants' eyes were opaque, obstructing the passage of light. Of 78 blinded infants, all but 10 of their mothers recalled having had German measles during the first three months of pregnancy. Gregg incriminated the rubella virus as the causative agent of the eye deformities in the newborn.

History repeated itself when a severe epidemic of rubella swept across Sweden in the spring of 1951 and across the United States in the early spring of 1964. The danger to the unborn child following rubella infection became manifestly evident. In the United States, there were approximately 20,000 blinded infants and unknown numbers of abortions and stillbirths. The birth of deformed infants was correlated with a positive history of rubella in nearly all their mothers.

The rubella virus has more than one effect on the infant. As well as being afflicted with cataract, many infants are born with malformed hearts, for the most part uncorrectable. Several suffer deafness, others are mentally retarded, and still others are microcephalic. The newborn infants are generally

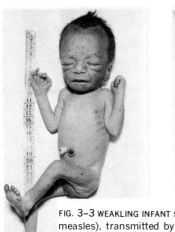 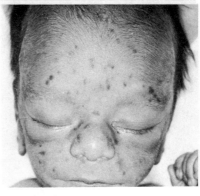

FIG. 3–3 WEAKLING INFANT suffering from congenital rubella (German measles), transmitted by the mother who had contracted German measles during pregnancy. (Courtesy of Dr. Arnold Rudolph, Baylor University School of Medicine, and with permission of the American Medical Association.)

stunted in growth; most of them weigh less than 5½ pounds and many less than 4½ pounds (FIG. 3-3).

The risk of damage to the fetus from maternal rubella is almost wholly during the first three months of pregnancy. The earlier in pregnancy the infection occurs, the greater the chances of injury to the infant. A study in 1960 by Drs. Richard H. Michaels and Gilbert W. Mellin of the Columbia University College of Physicians and Surgeons revealed that 47 to 50 percent of the newborn babies were abnormal if their mothers acquired the disease during the first month of pregnancy. The incidence of fetal defects decreased to 22 percent when maternal rubella occurred in the second month, and to 7 percent in the third month. After the third month of pregnancy, the risk of fetal malformations from maternal rubella is negligible.

In the years to come, rubella-damaged babies should be rare. In 1969, a vaccine, made from a weakened form of the live rubella virus, was successfully developed and marketed. The development of the vaccine began in 1961 when several investigators isolated the virus and devised the means of growing the virus in laboratory cultures. Subsequently, Drs. Paul D. Parkman and Harry M. Meyer, Jr., of the National Institutes of Health attenuated ("tamed") the virus so that in a vaccine, it would not cause the disease but would trigger the production of protective substances, or antibodies. Antibodies persist for years in the body and combat the virus if the person were to be exposed in later life to rubella infection. The person is said to develop an immunity against the disease.

With the hope of conferring immunity particularly to young girls before they reach the childbearing age, a campaign was launched in 1969 to vaccinate all children between the ages of one and seven. The mass inoculation of children is also intended to prevent widespread outbreaks of the disease, or at least reduce the spread of the disease—thus minimizing the risk of exposure of pregnant women to rubella infection.

Drugs and Viruses

THE EFFECTS OF thalidomide and the rubella virus on the fetus illustrate vividly that a harmful agent can cross the placenta and cause severe malformations, if the dosage and timing are appropriate. In recent years, numerous drugs and viruses have been suspected of having teratogenic properties in the human. Several medical researchers have reported congenital malformations in infants whose mothers had had mumps, chickenpox, smallpox, hepatitis, and other viral diseases during pregnancy. Developmental defects have been attributed to tranquilizing drugs taken by the pregnant mother, such as chloropromazine, meprobramate, and reserpine; to antibiotics and sulpha drugs; and to a host of other chemical substances and drugs, including aminopterin, folic acid, thiadiazole, meclizine, quinine, and salicylates (aspirin). Pregnant women, despite the thalidomide scare, are still consuming large quantities of drugs in the early part of their pregnancy. The pregnant mother today in the United States consumes an average of four drugs.

It is difficult, however, to assess the detrimental influences, if any, of the aforementioned viruses and drugs. None of the drugs listed above is known to affect such large numbers of infants as does thalidomide, nor do they produce a specific, rather unconventional defect such as phocomelia. If thalidomide had produced only a common disorder, such as hydrocephaly, which appeared only in a few infants, it probably would not have been suspected. In other words, the relationship between cause and effect is not apparent for most viruses and drugs since the deformities allegedly produced are indistinguishable from those commonly observed.

The controversy over the teratogenic potential of the influenza virus may be taken as a striking demonstration of the great uncertainty that exists. In the laboratory, it has been convincingly shown that chicken embryos, infected with influenza virus, develop severe malformations such as anencephaly and microcephaly. A high abortion rate has been witnessed in pregnant mice infected with a human strain of influenza virus. In humans, the relation of maternal influenza to fetal anomalies is far from clear. The pandemic of Asian influenza in 1957 provided an unusual opportunity for investigation. Most medical observers in the United States are agreed that there has been no significant increase in anomalies in infants born to pregnant mothers who have had Asian influenza. On the other hand, investigators in Ireland claim a substantial increase in fetal deformities attributable to Asian influenza. Still other investigators assert that the influenza virus leads to early widespread damage of the embryo, resulting in a high incidence of abortions and stillbirths. One cannot draw any valid conclusions, although it would be unwarranted to conclude at this time that influenza virus is not teratogenic in humans.

Antibiotics and sulpha drugs have given strong grounds for suspicion as teratogenic agents. All these therapeutic chemicals—penicillin, streptomycin, actinomycin D, terramycin, sulphanilamide, and sulphadiazine—pass through the placenta to the fetus. These drugs given to pregnant mice and rats have induced abortions and a diversity of fetal malformations involving damage to the eyes, brain, heart, and skeleton. There is yet no convincing evidence to suggest that these drugs are injurious to the human fetus.

Meclizine, an antihistamine widely used by pregnant women to overcome nausea, has been suspected of being teratogenic. Health authorities in Sweden forced the withdrawal of meclizine from public sale in 1961. Since that time a number of studies have failed to demonstrate any detrimental effects of meclizine on the embryo or fetus. Quinine, in large doses, has been taken early in pregnancy to stimulate an abortion. Where the abortion attempts have been unsuccessful, several infants have been born with brain damage and skeletal defects. It may well be that there is a strong association of malformed births and quinine intake by the mother. The obvious problem is the difficulty in obtaining reliable information on attempted abortions.

Insulin has long been known to cause fetal malformations when administered to pregnant rats, mice, and rabbits. In humans, it would appear that the diabetic mother, dependent on insulin, does not provide the most favorable uterine environment to her unborn infant. However, controversy continues to exist as to whether or not insulin crosses the placenta. It has been repeatedly observed that infants born to diabetic mothers tend to be large or overweight. The excessive size of such infants is thought to be related to enlargement and overactivity of the infant's pancreas. Several investigators have confirmed the fact that the pancreas of an infant of a diabetic mother secretes unusually large quantities of insulin. The extent to which this abnormal physiological condition is related to gross deformities is not evident. If gross abnormalities do occur, there is no specific pattern of deformity.

Ionizing Radiation

THE ADVENT of the atomic age has focused attention on the hazards to the fetus of high energy or ionizing radiation. Studies of the Japanese children whose mothers had been pregnant at the time of the atomic blasts at Hiroshima and Nagasaki reveal that several are now retarded in growth, microcephalic, and mentally deficient. These anomalies were probably the consequence of the irradiation, although statistically it cannot be demonstrated that the atomic explosions caused a significant increase in the incidence of fetal malformations. Notwithstanding the absence of rigorous documentation, it seems clear that irradiation of all types should be avoided when possible during pregnancy.

The view may be safely expressed that postconception irradiation is potentially hazardous to the fetus. An illuminating study was carried out in 1928 by Dr. Douglas P. Murphy and his co-workers at the Department of Obstetrics of the University of Pennsylvania. Among 74 newborn infants whose mothers had been administered therapeutic amounts of pelvic radium or X-ray irradiation during pregnancy, 38, or 50 percent, were abnormal. In 10 of these malformed infants, factors other than irradiation were implicated. In the remaining 28, the pelvic irradiation was judged to be the sole causative agent. Sixteen of the 28 infants were microcephalic idiots. This unusually high incidence of microcephaly constitutes strong presumptive evidence that the anomalies were radiation-induced. Other abnormalities observed included hydrocephaly, spina bifida, and clubfoot. The conclusion is inescapable that pelvic irradiation of pregnant mothers is extremely likely to be followed by the birth of a defective infant. The danger of irradiation is not only impairment of the bodily structures of the fetus, but also damage to the hereditary units (the genes) in the germinal tissues of the gonads of the mother and child.

Whereas radiation-induced body anomalies are not passed on to the next generation, radiation-induced defective genes can be transmitted to subsequent generations. Indeed, the concealed genetic damage can be considerable.

General Principles in Teratogenesis

CERTAIN GENERALIZATIONS have emerged from the studies of teratogenic agents in experimental animals and the observations of fetal anomalies in humans. It has become increasingly clear that drugs, or viruses, or X rays may have little or no detrimental effect on the mother and yet may be disastrous to the fetus. This violates the cherished belief that the uterine environment provided by the mother is an impenetrable haven for her unborn child.

The particular type of fetal malformation is related to the time in development at which the noxious agent is administered or becomes active. Certain deleterious agents, when applied at specific developmental stages, produce characteristic patterns of abnormality. We have seen, for example, that the anomalies resulting from thalidomide have a specific pattern, and that the sensitive period of development is between the 35th and the 50th day of pregnancy. The sensitivity of an organ to a teratogenic influence is greatest during a limited developmental period when the organ or part is undergoing rapid differentiation or growth. Since the major structuring of the organs of the infant occurs during the first three months of pregnancy, it is understandable that the unborn child is especially vulnerable during this developmental period. It may be recalled that the risk of damage to the embryo from maternal German measles is negligible after the third month of pregnancy.

Another well-established fact is that a given teratogen produces different malformations when applied at different times of development. X rays cause primarily fetal defects of the eye and brain when administered to pregnant rats on the ninth day of gestation, but cause mainly skeletal defects in the fetus when given on the 14th day. Moreover, different teratogens acting during the same period of development may affect different phases of the developmental process. The two agents, thalidomide and rubella virus, produce entirely different defects by exerting their effects on different developmental pathways.

Investigators have also been quick to notice that the patterns of abnormalities may be quite different in different species of animals. Thus, when pregnant rats are fed a diet deficient in vitamin A, the offspring are typically hydrocephalic. On the other hand, mice maintained on diets deficient in vitamin A during pregnancy produce offspring with ocular, genital, and kidney defects. Thalidomide in humans is a violent teratogen; yet, on testing with a wide variety of laboratory animals, it has proved to be relatively innocuous. The wide variability of response of different species prompted Dr. Allan C. Barnes of the Johns Hopkins School of Medicine to remark in 1968 that "the only test for teratogenicity in man is man himself."

Finally, and perhaps most importantly, the potential deleterious effect of a teratogen is influenced by the genetic constitution of the organism. The work of the Canadian geneticist F. Clarke Fraser and his colleagues at McGill University in Montreal has made it abundantly clear that a fetal defect is a consequence of an interplay of genetic factors and environmental influences.

Interplay of Genes and Environment

IN 1957, DR. FRASER AND his co-workers contributed convincing evidence that the action of an environmental agent is influenced by the genetic constitution of the animal. Cleft palate can be induced in mouse embryos by treating the pregnant mothers with cortisone (FIG. 3–4). Cortisone is a hormone normally secreted by the adrenal gland and, parenthetically, a substance much used to relieve sufferers of arthritis.

One genetic strain of mice (strain A) is particularly susceptible to cortisone-induced cleft palate. A prescribed dose of cortisone administered at an early stage of gestation causes cleft palate in 100 percent of the offspring of strain A (FIG. 3–5, cross 1). It was then found that the same treatment given to pregnant females of another genetically different strain (strain B) produced cleft palate in only 19 percent of the offspring (FIG. 3–5, cross 2). When females of strain A were crossed with

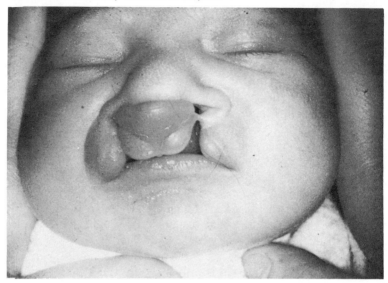

FIG. 3-4 CLEFT PALATE, a break or opening in the bony structure that supports the upper part of the mouth. (Courtesy of Dr. Norman Woody, Tulane University School of Medicine.)

males of strain B, the cortisone-treated mothers produced hybrid offspring of which 43 percent had cleft palates (FIG. 3-5, cross 3). This was not unexpected, since hybrid offspring are often intermediate between the parental strains. But, in the reciprocal cross involving B mothers and A fathers, the incidence of cleft palate among these hybrid offspring of cortisone-treated mothers was only four percent (FIG. 3-5, cross 4). It should thus be obvious that the probability that an embryo will develop cleft palate is strongly influenced by the mother's uterine environment. The hybrid embryo growing in the womb of an A mother (cross 3) is more subject to damage than the same hybrid offspring growing in the womb of a B mother (cross 4). At the same time, the probability of cleft palate relates to the genetic makeup of the embryos. It is to be noted that the genetically different embryos of crosses 1 and 3, although both growing in A mothers, have different frequencies of cleft palate. Likewise, embryos of crosses 2 and 4 differ in the incidence of cleft palate, even though both were carried by mothers of similar genetic constitutions (strain B).

It is clear, then, that individuals of different genetic constitutions may respond to the same teratogenic agent to differing degrees. The vast majority of malformations are not the result of a single genetic factor or a single external agent, but of a complicated interaction of many genetic factors and many environmental factors. The human geneticist James V. Neel postulates that approximately 20 percent of all congenital anomalies result from major defective genes with relatively

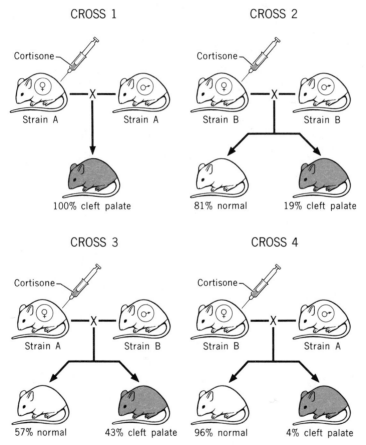

FIG. 3–5 LABORATORY CROSSES of two different strains of mice reveal the interplay of genetic factors and environmental influences in the development and incidence of cleft palate. (Based on studies by Dr. Clarke Fraser, McGill University, Montreal, Canada.)

simple inheritance patterns. In these cases, discussed in Chapter 4, the genetic effects are scarcely tempered by environmental influences. Not more than 10 percent of the total can be accounted for by mishaps in chromosome numbers, an intriguing phenomenon that will be treated in Chapters 5 and 6. An additional 10 percent results from the action of very specific agents, such as thalidomide, in which the genetic constitution of the mother or the fetus does not appear to play a modulating role. The remaining 60 percent represents the disruption of developmental pathways occasioned by the interaction of complex genetic systems and relatively minor environmental fluctuations. Stated another way, an hereditary predisposition which might otherwise not reveal itself may be triggered to produce a malformation by subtle adverse factors in the uterine environment.

The unborn child has no control over the genes transmitted to it by the parents, nor for that matter over the environment furnished it by the mother. In a very large sense, the fetus inherits *both* genes and an environment.

You would think, that with all the possible environmental factors which are potentially teratogenic, there would be more genetic malformation.

Chapter 4

Gene-Associated Defects

OUR PRESENT KNOWLEDGE of heredity rests on certain principles discovered through the painstaking work of the humble Austrian monk Gregor Johann Mendel (1822–1884). No discovery in the field of biology has had more impact or is more far-reaching in importance than the formulation of the fundamental laws of inheritance by Mendel. Ironically, Mendel's monumental paper, published in 1866, was overlooked by most scientists of the day. His important contribution lay ignored or unknown until 1900, sixteen years after his death. Since the turn of the century, extensive studies have added to and extended Mendel's findings. An indisputable fact that has emerged is that the laws of inheritance are equally valid for all kinds of living things, including man himself.

The organisms favored for study by geneticists are those which can be grown experimentally in large numbers and which breed rapidly. The fruit fly, mold, wheat, and corn admirably meet these qualifications. Humans, obviously, are not ideal subjects for genetical investigation. The accepted social institution of monogamy, the comparatively long life of the individual, the one child at birth, and the relatively few children born to the parents, are all limiting factors in the study of human inheritance. In the absence of direct experimentation on humans, the geneticist must content himself with marriages that have already taken place. The analysis of family histories is understandably less precise than controlled breeding experiments in the laboratory. Nevertheless, substantial and invaluable information has accumulated through the careful analysis of a very large number of human pedigrees.

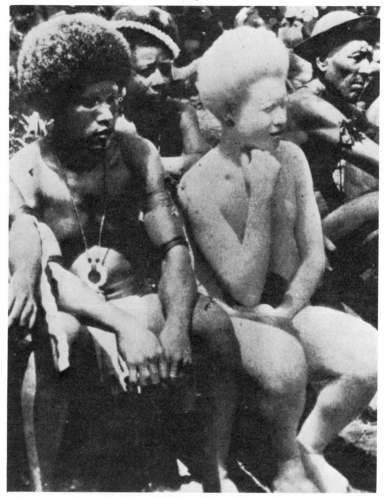

FIG. 4-1 ALBINO PERSON showing the complete absence of pigment in the eyes, hair, and skin. (From the *Journal of Heredity* 39: 131, 1948.)

Simple Mendelian Principles

THE UNITS OF HEREDITY, or genes, occur in pairs in the fertilized egg. The newborn infant inherits one gene of each pair from the mother and one of each pair from the father. It is a cardinal fact that each transmissible trait is governed by at least one pair of genes. The human geneticist draws conclusions about the kinds of genes from the presence of certain traits in the infant, the parents, and relatives.

Albinism in man may be taken as an illustrative example of a trait under the simple control of a single pair of genes. Albinism occurs among all racial groups (FIG. 4-1), but at different frequencies in various human populations. Its highest incidence is among the San Blas Indians of central Panama, where as many as seven infants per thousand are reported to be albinos. In France and Russia, about one person in 100,000 is albino, while in the United States the frequency increases to one person in 10,000. The world-wide incidence of albinism is about one in 20,000.

The word "albino" is derived from the Latin *albus,* meaning white, and refers to the absence of pigment in the skin, hair, and eyes. The skin is often very light ("milk–white"), and the hair whitish–yellow. The eyes appear pinkish because the red blood vessels give the otherwise colorless iris a rosy cast. Albinos have poor vision and are acutely sensitive to sunlight. They are extremely prone to skin cancer.

Albinism results from a defective gene. Specifically, the condition arises only when the individual is endowed with two defective genes, one from each parent. It is important to remember that the affected person must have received the defective gene for albinism from both parents.

As seen in FIGURE 4-2, there are nine possible marriages with respect to the pair of genes conditioning the presence or absence of pigment in man. If both parents are perfectly normal—that is, each carries a pair of normal genes—then all offspring will be normal (cross 1). When both parents are albino and accordingly each carries a pair of defective genes, all offspring will be afflicted with albinism (cross 2). The persons involved in either of these two crosses are said to be *homozygous,* since they each carry a pair of similar, or like, genes. The normal individuals in cross 1 are homozygous for the normal gene, and the albino individuals in cross 2 are homozygous for the defective gene.

Turning our attention to cross 3, we notice that one of the parents (the mother) carries an unlike pair of genes: one member of the pair is normal and its partner gene is defective. This

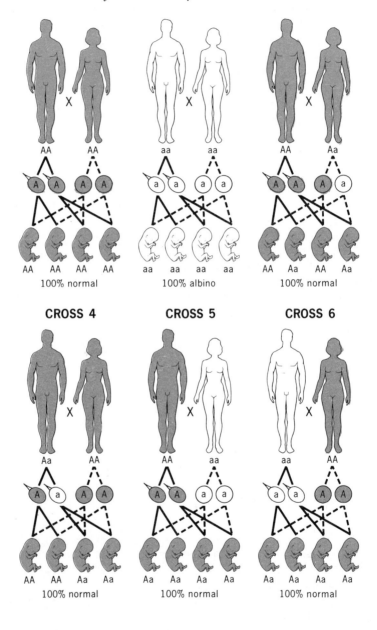

AA   AA
100% normal

aa   aa
100% albino

AA   Aa
100% normal

CROSS 4   **CROSS 5**   **CROSS 6**

Aa   AA
AA   AA   Aa   Aa
100% normal

AA   aa
Aa   Aa   Aa   Aa
100% normal

aa   AA
Aa   Aa   Aa   Aa
100% normal

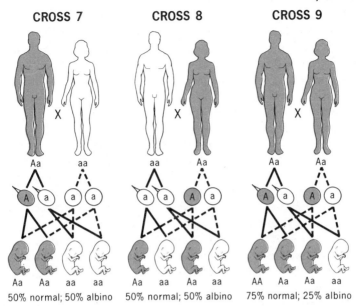

CROSS 7   **CROSS 8**   **CROSS 9**

FIG. 4–2 OUTCOME of nine possible marriages involving a recessive trait, such as albinism. Affected offspring receive the defective recessive gene (designated *a*) from both parents.

parent, carrying unlike genes, is *heterozygous.* This parent has normal coloration, which leads us to deduce that the expression of the defective gene is completely masked or suppressed by the normal gene. In genetical parlance, we say that the normal gene is *dominant* over its partner, the recessive gene. The dominant gene is customarily symbolized by a capital letter (in our case, *A);* the recessive gene, by a corresponding small letter *(a).* The heterozygous parent may be depicted as *Aa,* and may be referred to as a *heterozygote* or a *carrier.*

When the heterozygote *(Aa)* marries the dominant homozygote *(AA),* all the offspring will be outwardly normal, but half the offspring will be carriers *(Aa)* like one of the parents (cross 3). Cross 4 differs from cross 3 only in that the father is the carrier *(Aa)* and the mother is the dominant homozygote *(AA).* The outcome is the same: all children are normal in appearance but half of them are carriers. Thus, with respect to albinism, the males and females are equally likely to have or to transmit the trait. In a later chapter, we will learn of traits in which transmission is influenced by the sex of the parents.

All offspring will be carriers from the marriage (crosses 5 and 6) of a dominant homozygote *(AA)* and an albino parent *(aa)*. Examining crosses 5 and 6 (FIG. 4–2), we notice, once again, that males and females are equally likely to be affected. The marriage of a heterozygous person *(Aa)* and an albino *(aa)* gives rise to two types of progeny, in equal numbers (crosses 7 and 8). Half the offspring are normal but carriers *(Aa);* the remaining half are albino *(aa)*.

Another cardinal fact of inheritance is that each gamete (egg or sperm) contains *one and only one* member of a pair of genes. Thus, when the egg and sperm unite, the two genes for each character are brought back together in the new individual. During the production of the sex cells, the members of a pair of genes separate, or *segregate,* from each other. A given gamete can carry *A* or *a,* but not both. This fundamental concept that only one member of any pair of genes in a parent is transmitted to each offspring is known as Mendel's *Law of Segregation.*

The foregoing knowledge permits an appreciation of the outcome of the last of the crosses (no. 9) depicted in FIGURE 4–2. Both parents are normal in appearance, but each carries the defective gene *(a)* masked by the normal gene *(A)*. The male parent produces two kinds of sperm cells: half the sperm carry the *A* gene and half carry the *a* gene. The same two kinds occur in equal proportions among the egg cells. Each kind of sperm has an equal chance of meeting each kind of egg. The random meeting of gametes leads to both normal and albino offspring. One-quarter of the progeny are normal and completely devoid of the recessive gene *(AA);* one-half are normal but carriers, like the parents *(Aa);* and the remaining one quarter exhibit the albino anomaly *(aa)*. There are three genetically different types of offspring, or technically, three different *genotypes: AA, Aa, aa.* The ratio of genotypes may be expressed as 1/4 *AA:* 1/2 *Aa:* 1/4 *aa,* or simply 1:2:1. The dominant homozygote *(AA)* can not be distinguished by inspection from the heterozygote *(Aa)*. In genetic terminology, we say that the *AA* and *Aa* genotypes have the same *phenotype* (same external or observable appearance). Thus, on the basis of phenotype alone, the progeny ratio is 3/4 normal: 1/4 albino, or 3:1.

If we disregard the sex of the parents, the nine crosses in FIGURE 4–2 become reducible to six possible types of marriages. The six kinds of marriages involving a single pair of genes are set forth in TABLE 4–1.

Normal and Recessive Offspring

IT SHOULD BE UNDERSTOOD that the 3:1 phenotypic ratio resulting from the marriage of two heterozygotes, or the 1:1 ratio from the marriage of a heterozygote and a recessive person, are expectations based on probability. The production of large numbers of progeny increases the probability of obtaining, for example, the 1:1 progeny ratio, just as many tosses of a coin improve the chances of approximating the expected 1 "head": 1 "tail" ratio. If a coin is tossed only two times a "head" on the first toss is not invariably followed by a "tail" on the second toss. In like manner, if only two offspring are produced from the marriage of heterozygous and recessive parents, it should not be thought that one normal offspring is always accompanied by one recessive offspring. With small numbers of progeny, as is characteristic in man, any ratio

TABLE 4–1

Simple Recessive Mendelian Inheritance
Single Pair of Genes (Normal Pigmentation vs. Albinism)

Marriages		Gametes		Offspring	
Genotypes	Phenotypes	First parent	Second parent	Genotypes	Phenotypes
		50% 50%	50% 50%		
$AA \times AA$	normal × normal	A A	A A	100% AA	100% normal
$AA \times Aa$	normal × normal	A A	A a	50% AA 50% Aa	100% normal
$Aa \times Aa$	normal × normal	A a	A a	25% AA 50% Aa 25% aa	75% normal 25% albino
$AA \times aa$	normal × albino	A A	a a	100% Aa	100% normal
$Aa \times aa$	normal × albino	A a	a a	50% AA 50% aa	50% normal 50% albino
$aa \times aa$	albino × albino	a a	a a	100% aa	100% albino

might arise in a given family. Stated another way, the 3:1 and 1:1 ratios reveal the risks or odds of a given child having the particular trait involved. If the first child of two heterozygous parents is an albino, the odds that the second child will be an albino remains 1 out of 4. These odds hold for each subsequent child, irrespective of the number of previously affected children. Each birth is an entirely independent event.

Recessively Inherited Disorders

IN THE VAST MAJORITY of cases of recessive inheritance, affected persons are derived from marriages of two heterozygous carriers. In other words, recessive disorders tend to appear only among siblings, not in their parents. This is exemplified by the family pedigree in FIGURE 4–3. In the diagram shown, a square indicates a male (identified also by the symbol of Mars, ♂); a circle denotes a female (represented also by the symbol of Venus, ♀). The hollow or unshaded symbol denotes a normal person, and the shaded or solid symbol represents a person afflicted with the disorder. A marriage between two individuals is indicated by a horizontal line con-

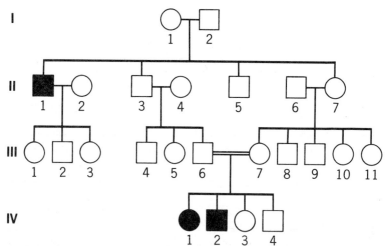

FIG. 4–3 PEDIGREE OF A RECESSIVELY INHERITED DISORDER, involving a marriage of cousins. The marriage of near relatives increases the risk that both partners have received the same detrimental recessive gene through a common ancestor.

necting their symbols; consanguineous marriages involving close relatives are represented by two horizontal lines. Successive generations are designated by Roman numerals, while the various individuals within a generation are numbered consecutively, from left to right, with Arabic figures.

FIGURE 4-3 states, in symbolic form, that a normal man marries a normal woman. Apparently, both were heterozygous carriers since one of the four children (the first child, designated II-1) exhibited the recessive trait. This son, although affected, had three normal offspring (III—1, -2, and -3). These three children must be carriers *(Aa),* having received the *a* gene from their father, and the *A* gene from the unaffected mother (II-2). The genetic constitution of the mother (II-2) can not be ascertained; she may be either homozygous dominant *(AA)* or a heterozygous carrier *(Aa).*

We can also deduce that the daughter (II-7) of the first marriage was a carrier *(Aa).* All her children were normal, but it is to be noted that her first child (III-7) married a first cousin (III-6), from which marriage were born affected children (IV-1 and -2). Accordingly, the daughter of the third generation (III-7) must have been heterozygous, and, in turn, her mother (II-7) was most likely heterozygous (unless she happened to marry a heterozygous man). Similarly, the male involved in the consanguineous marriage (III-6) must have been heterozygous.

Special significance is attached to the heterozygous carrier—the individual who carries the recessive gene entirely unsuspected. It is usually impossible to tell, prior to the marriage, whether the individual bears the detrimental recessive gene. Thus, the recessive gene may be transmitted without any outward manifestation for several generations, continually being sheltered by the dominant normal gene. The recessive gene, however, does become exposed when two carrier parents happen to mate, as we have seen in FIGURE 4-3. This explains cases in which a trait absent for many generations can suddenly appear without warning. Often only one member in a family is afflicted. In such an event, it would be an error to jump to the conclusion that the abnormality is not hereditary solely because there are no other cases in the family.

Offspring afflicted with a recessive disorder tend to arise

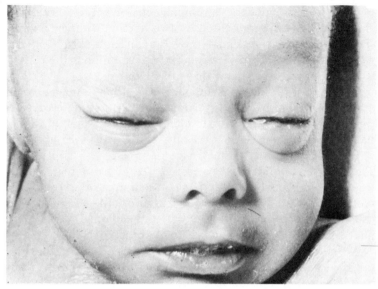

FIG. 4-4 CONGENITAL ICHTHYOSIS, a lethal recessive disorder characterized by extreme dryness of the skin. Infants with this disorder rarely survive beyond a week. (Courtesy of Dr. Norman Woody, Tulane University School of Medicine.)

more often from consanguineous unions than from marriages of unrelated persons. Close relatives share more of the same genes than persons from the population at large. If a recessive trait is extremely rare, the chance is very small that unrelated marriage partners will both harbor the same defective gene. The marriage of close relatives, however, increases the risk that both partners have received the same defective gene through some common ancestor.

Lethal Recessive Inheritance

SOMETIMES A RECESSIVE GENE is so drastic in its effect that nothing can be done to save the life of the infant or prolong his life to maturity. There are several examples in man of fatal, or lethal, recessive genes. One lethal disorder is congenital ichthyosis, characterized by the cracking and separation of the skin into large scaly sections (FIG. 4–4). Infants carrying a double dose of the recessive gene for ichthyosis are generally aborted or born prematurely. Those managing to survive birth die in about three days. There is no therapy for this severe anomaly.

Another fatal inherited condition is infantile amaurotic idiocy. It is also known as Tay-Sachs disease, after its co-discoverers, the British ophthalmologist Warren Tay (1843–1927) and the American neurologist Bernard P. Sachs (1858–1944). Affected children appear normal and healthy at birth, but within six months the nerves of the brain and spinal cord exhibit marked signs of deterioration. At first listless and irritable, the infant finds it increasingly difficult to sit up or stand. By the age of one year, the child lies helplessly in his crib. He becomes mentally retarded, progressively blind, and finally paralyzed. The disease takes its lethal toll by the age of three to four years. There are no known survivors and no cure.

A feature of special interest is that nine out of 10 affected children are of Jewish heritage. It is especially common in Jews of northeastern European origin, particularly from provinces in Lithuania and Poland. In the United States, Tay-Sachs disease is about a hundred times more prevalent in the Jewish population than among non-Jews. The frequency of heterozygous carriers has been estimated at one in 45 for Jews and one in 350 for non-Jews. The factors responsible for the exceptionally elevated incidence of the disease in the Jewish population remain puzzling.

One of the most devastating recessive disorders among children is cystic fibrosis of the pancreas. About 6,000 infants are born with the disease each year in the United States. There are at least five million heterozygous carriers, and one child in every thousand is born with the disease. Virtually all infants with cystic fibrosis are Caucasians; Negroes and Orientals are rarely afflicted.

Less than 35 years ago, cystic fibrosis was not even recognized as a distinct entity. Today it has the unenviable reputation of being one of the most important disorders of childhood. Intestinal obstruction is the first symptom of the disease; the infant's stools are frequent, large, and foul. The pancreas secretes a mucous material that is abnormally thick or viscid, with the consequence that digestion is blocked in the intestinal tract. All mucous-secreting tissues are abnormal. The sticky mucus produced by the lungs is particularly serious; the lungs become clogged and the child has repeated bouts of pneumonia. A characteristic finding, by which cystic fibrosis is most readily diagnosed, is the increased amount of salt in the sweat.

Before the introduction of antibiotics, affected children invariably died in infancy of constant infection. New drugs, inhaled as vapor, soften the thick mucus of the lungs and have enabled some children to weather the difficult first years. The widespread application of antibiotics has led to a considerable reduction in early mortality. A few patients have survived to reproduce.

Disorders of Dominant Inheritance

THE FAMILY PEDIGREE shown in FIGURE 4-5 has certain intriguing features. It may be noted that each affected person has at least one affected parent. Moreover, the normal children of an affected parent, when they in turn marry normal persons, have only normal offspring. In this particular instance, the harmful gene is dominant and the normal gene is recessive. In nearly all instances of dominant inheritance, as exemplified by the pedigree, one parent carries the harmful gene and shows the anomaly, whereas the other parent is normal. The affected parent will pass on the defective dominant gene, on the average, to 50 percent of the children. The normal children

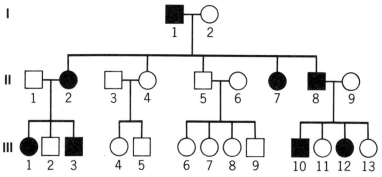

FIG. 4-5 PEDIGREE OF DOMINANT INHERITANCE, showing that the dominant disorder is transmitted only by those individuals who display the disorder and never by unaffected individuals. Solid symbol represents a person afflicted with the disorder; unshaded symbol denotes an unaffected person.

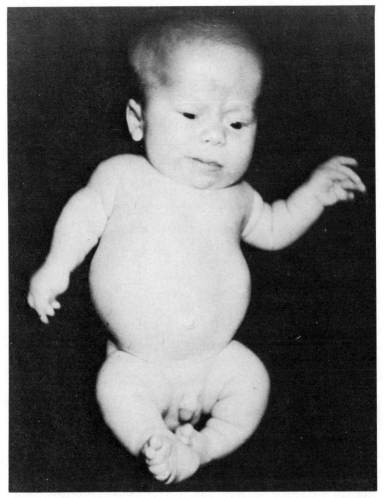

FIG. 4-6 ACHONDROPLASTIC DWARFISM, a dominant genetic disorder in which the child has inherited abnormally short arms and legs. (Courtesy of Dr. Norman Woody, Tulane University School of Medicine.)

do not carry the abnormal dominant gene, and hence their offspring and further descendants are not burdened with the dominant trait.

There are numerous examples in man of defective genes that are transmitted in a dominant pattern. Achondroplasia, a form of dwarfism, is always dominant in man. Affected individuals

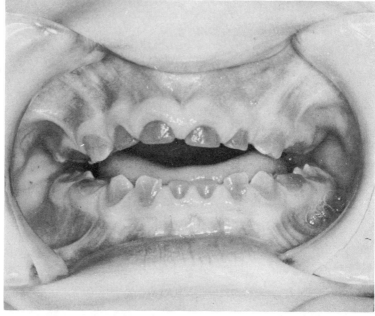

FIG. 4-7 DISFIGURING DOMINANT TRAIT in which the teeth are discolored and the crowns are markedly worn down. (From J. S. Thompson and M. W. Thompson, *Genetics in Medicine*, W. B. Saunders, Philadelphia, 1966.)

are small and disproportionate, with abnormally short arms and legs (FIG. 4-6). The defect is evident at birth, and most achondroplastic dwarfs fail to survive beyond the first year. Only about 20 percent of the affected individuals reach adulthood.

Other examples of dominant traits are tylosis, a condition in which the skin of the palms and soles is excessively thickened; anonychia, a condition in which some or all of the nails of the fingers and toes are absent; and dentinogenesis imperfecta, a disorder in which the crowns of teeth wear down readily (FIG. 4-7). Two relatively common dominant defects are polydactyly (extra fingers or toes) and brachydactyly (FIG. 4-8); the hands of brachydactylous persons are short, stocky, and thick. There is a shortening of both the fingers and palms. In sharp contrast, persons afflicted with Marfan's syndrome have unusually long, or tapering, fingers (FIG. 4-8). Patients with Marfan's syndrome have poor musculature and long, thin extremities. Some medical authorities believe that Abraham Lincoln, who was exceptionally long-limbed, suffered from this dominant disorder.

Dominant defects that are not of a very serious nature may be transmitted through many generations. The more severe dominant anomalies are incompatible with reproduction and accordingly are not transmitted at all. There is, however, one way in which a very serious dominant disorder can be handed on through many generations. Transmission can take place if the anomaly does not manifest itself until comparatively late in life, after the affected person has already had children.

An unfortunate example of such a late-appearing dominant defect is Huntington's chorea, characterized by disorganized muscular movements and progressive mental deterioration. The disease shows itself between the ages of 25 and 55. A parent may die before the defect manifests itself—but only after the parent may have transmitted the condition to his

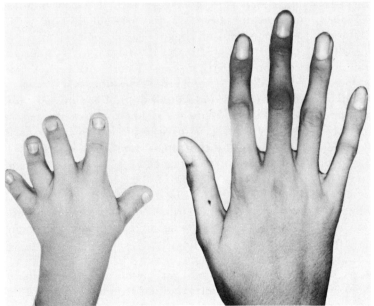

FIG. 4-8 SHARP CONTRASTS in the hands of persons afflicted with brachydactyly (short fingers) and Marfan's syndrome (long, tapering fingers). (*Left,* From D. Hoefnagel and P. S. Gerald, *Annals of Human Genetics* 29: 377-382, 1966; *Right* Courtesy of Dr. Norman Woody, Tulane University School of Medicine.)

offspring. Each child of a choreic parent has a 1:1 chance to be afflicted in later life like his parent. As an individual from an afflicted family passes the age of 55 without manifesting the disorder, he can have increasing assurance that his children will be free of the disorder.

Huntington's chorea is sufficiently common to provide two or three cases at any one time at the average large mental hospital. The marriage rate and fertility of choreic persons are both high. The average choreic family has about five children. This shows the perversity of the human race in the face of evident dangers.

Defective Genes and Mutation

CAN A DETRIMENTAL GENE be eradicated from the population of man? Let us return to the recessive condition of albinism. Albinism is exceedingly rare. It has been estimated that one out of 20,000 individuals are albino. It may be thought that most albino children come from marriages of two homozygous albinos. This is not true. The great majority of affected children—more than 99 percent—come from marriages of two normally pigmented, but heterozygous, parents.

Heterozygous, or carrier, individuals are not as rare as might be supposed. Indeed, the frequency of heterozygous carriers is many times greater than that of recessive albino individuals. Reliable estimates indicate that approximately 1.4 percent of all individuals, or one out of 70 persons, are carriers of the albino gene. In other words, there are 280 times as many carriers as affected individuals. The fact that heterozygous carriers cannot be distinguished from normal homozygotes or noncarriers militates against any scheme aimed at eliminating an undesirable genetic trait in man.

Many albino individuals do not survive to adulthood, fail to marry, or produce fewer offspring than normal. Since albino individuals have great mortality and low fecundity, it might be expected that the abnormal gene for albinism would pass rapidly from existence, or at least steadily decrease from one generation to the next. Each failure of a homozygous albino individual to transmit his genes would result each time in the loss of two defective recessive genes from the population. Yet the albino gene has not decreased in frequency!

The factor that maintains the albino gene in the population is *mutation*. A mutation is an alteration in the normal gene. A mishap occurs in the normal copying process of the gene. New mutations arise from time to time, and the same mutations may occur repeatedly. In fact, all genes undergo mutation at some definable rate. In each generation, it can be expected that a certain proportion of normal genes will be converted, for example, into defective albino genes. Thus, while in every generation a large number of albino genes are lost from the population by the inability of albinos to leave descendants, this same number is replaced by the process of mutation. As long as the rate of elimination of the albino gene equals its rate of origin by mutation, the incidence of albinism in the human population will not change. Such a population is said to be in *genetic equilibrium* with respect to the albino gene.

An analogy shown in FIGURE 4-9A will help to visualize the concept of genetic equilibrium. The water level in the beaker remains constant when the rate at which water enters the opening of the beaker equals the rate at which it leaves the hole in the side of the beaker. In other words, a state of genetic equilibrium (constant water level in beaker) is reached when the rate at which the recessive gene is replenished by

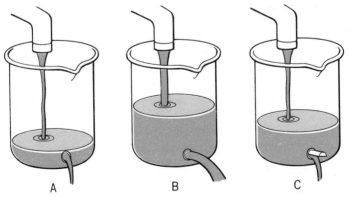

FIG. 4-9 INTERPLAY of detrimental mutant genes (water from faucet) and their elimination (water escaping through hole) in a human population (beaker) containing a reservoir of the harmful genes (water in beaker). See text for explanations.'

mutation (water from faucet) equals the rate at which it is lost through failure of reproduction of affected individuals (water leaving beaker).

What would be the consequences of an increase in the mutation rate? Man today lives in an environment in which high energy radiation is assuredly not calculated to improve the human germ plasm. In 1927, Hermann J. Muller (Nobel Laureate in Medicine, 1946) announced that genes are highly susceptible to the action of X rays. The process of mutation is enormously speeded up as the dosage of X rays increases. The ever-increasing ionizing radiation produced by fallout from atomic explosions has unquestionably induced many mutations. The consequence is shown in FIGURE 4-9*B*. The increased rate of mutation resulting from high energy radiation may be conceived as an increased input of water. The water level in the beaker will rise and water will escape more rapidly through the hole in the side of the beaker. Similarly, defective genes will be found more frequently in the population and will be eliminated at a faster rate from the population. A balance will be restored eventually between input and output; however, the population will then have a larger store of defective genes. Physicians in years to come will be called upon to treat a greater number of defective infants.

The supply of defective genes in the human population has already increased through the greater medical control of genetic disorders. The outstanding advances in modern medicine have served to prolong the lives of genetically defective persons who might otherwise not have survived to reproductive age. This may be compared to partially plugging the hole in the side of the beaker (FIG. 4-9*C)*. The water level in the beaker will obviously rise, as will the amount of defective genes in the population. There can be no loftier motive in society than to save lives by the application of medical knowledge. *But the price of our humanitarian principles is the enlargement of our pool of harmful genes and an increased incidence of genetically malformed infants.*

Chapter 5

Fetal Malformations of Chromosomal Origin

IN THE EARLY 1950's, the University of Iowa biologist Emil Witschi prepared a manuscript for a distinguished medical journal on a seemingly unconventional subject. The unusual topic concerned the fate of old, or "overripe," eggs deposited by female frogs. Ordinarily a female frog will release her mature eggs—1,000 or more—within a remarkably short span of time, a matter of several minutes. These freshly deposited eggs, when inseminated by the male, develop into perfectly normal embryos, the familiar polliwogs. Only freshly deposited eggs are capable of developing in a normal fashion. If the mature eggs remain too long (four or five days) in the body cavity of the female before being released, the eggs suffer degenerative changes, or, as we say, the eggs become aged or "overripe." The aged eggs can be fertilized but they are fated to grow into malformed, grotesquely shaped embryos.

The types of abnormalities which arise from overripe fertilized eggs are strangely reminiscent of the kinds of deformities occasionally witnessed in human embryos. The lower body region of the frog embryo may be severed in two parts, comparable to the anomaly in humans termed "spina bifida," in which the spinal cord is split at its lowest portion. The deformed frog embryo may have a tiny, or microcephalic, head or even be acephalic (headless). Double monsters are not uncommon among embryos from an overripe batch of eggs. These double monsters resemble the congenitally united Siamese twins in man.

A startling finding by Witschi was that the malformed frog embryos possess peculiar numbers of chromosomes within their cells. Chromosomes, you will recall, are the threadlike structures in the nucleus of the cell that carry the information of heredity. A normal organism has a characteristic number of chromosomes within each body cell, which in the frog happens to be 26. The defective embryos from the overripe eggs contain odd numbers of chromosomes, ranging from as few as 13 to as many as 52. FIGURE 5-1 shows the appearance of a grossly deformed embryo that has 25 chromosomes, one less than the normal number. The embryo has a distorted head, a curved body, and a defective tail. It is quite evident that a frog embryo cannot develop normally unless it has a full complement of chromosomes, and, furthermore, that overripeness of eggs is associated with faulty chromosome numbers.

One might be inclined to complacently dismiss these observations on the frog as interesting but esoteric, without significance for man. It may scarcely seem possible that congenital defects in humans could be linked to mishaps in the chromosomes of an individual. But in 1959, three French scientists at the University of Paris surprised the medical world with their announcement that a well-known human malformation was in fact associated with a chromosomal abnormality. Their discovery, received initially with some skepticism but now

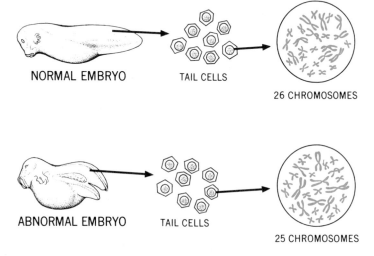

FIG. 5-1 SHARP CONTRAST in the features of frog embryos associated with different chromosome numbers. The abnormal embryo was derived from an old, or "overripe," egg, and has a faulty chromosome complement (25 chromosomes instead of the usual 26). The normal embryo has the proper number of chromosomes (26).

universally accepted, was made on mentally retarded children with small slanting eyes, the "mongoloid idiots."

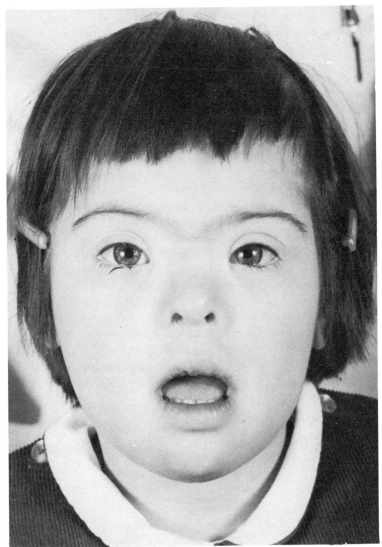

FIG. 5–2 FACIAL FEATURES of a 3½-year-old girl afflicted with mongolism. (From M. Bartalos and T. A. Baramski, *Medical Cytogenetics*, The Williams & Wilkins Co., Baltimore, 1967.)

Mongolism (Down's Syndrome)

DR. JOHN LANGDON DOWN (1828–1896), an eminent London physician, is remembered in medicine as the man who provided, in 1866, the first comprehensive description of mongolism. This congenital disability is unmistakably marked on the afflicted child's face: a prominent forehead, a flattened nasal bridge, an habitually open mouth, a projecting lower lip, a large protruding tongue, and a skin fold (epicanthic fold) at the inner corners of the eyes (FIG. 5-2). Dr. Down unjustifiably seized upon the Oriental-like cast of the eye to designate the disorder "mongoloid idiocy." This unwarranted expression and allied ones, like "mongolism," "mongolian idiot," and "mongol," tend to cast aspersions upon Oriental peoples. It is difficult, however, to obliterate these unfortunate names as they have become entrenched in the medical literature and have persisted in the popular mind. Medical scientists today have proposed to call the disorder "Down's syndrome," a term which is rapidly gaining acceptance and use. Irrespective of the terminology employed, the important consideration is the recognition that affected children bear no true resemblance to Mongolian peoples (unless they happen to be born among them). The eye folds of the afflicted child only superficially resemble the characteristic folds of Oriental persons (FIG. 5-3).

Down's syndrome is essentially a condition of arrested development, for which no cure has been discovered. Affected children were described by one imaginative writer in 1886 as "unfinished" and by another in 1907 as "ill-finished." These remarks were made in reference to the underdeveloped brain

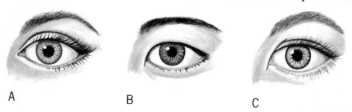

A   B   C

FIG. 5–3 MEDICAL BLUNDER in the description of the eye folds of the so-called "mongoloid" patient. The mongoloid patient has a distinct skin fold in the inner corner of the eye (C). The eye of the Oriental person is distinguished by a curved, overlapping eyelid (B). Except for the skin fold, the eye of the mongoloid patient is formed in the same way as that of any Caucasian person (A).

and poor muscular coordination of the mongoloid child. The tragic consequence of malformation of the brain is mental retardation. The majority of mongoloids are imbeciles, rather than idiots, with intelligence quotients between 25 and 49. Dr. Benjamin Malzberg's elaborate study in the 1950's on the intelligence levels of 880 mongoloid children in the New York State schools showed that 24 percent were idiots (IQ less than 25), 72 percent were imbeciles (IQ between 25 and 49), and 4 percent were morons (IQ between 50 and 69). The cheerful and gregarious disposition of the mongoloid child, together with his strong powers of mimicry and love of music, makes him appear more intelligent than he is. Less than four per 100 are able to read with comprehension, and only two per 100 ever learn to write. As infants, mongoloids are retarded in their capacity to sit, stand, and walk. Whereas normal infants begin to walk at the age of 12 months, most mongoloids do not learn to walk until two to three years of age. Their movements remain slow and clumsy throughout life.

Mongoloid children are incapable of caring for themselves and must always remain dependent on others. Mongoloids account for about 15 percent of the inmates of institutions for mental defectives in the United States. There has been a growing tendency to institutionalize mongol children, despite various findings which support the conclusion that home-cared mongoloid children are superior in both social and physical development than those confined in institutions at birth.

The heart is malformed in many of the afflicted children. Estimates indicate that between 40 and 60 percent have serious heart defects. Of those that have heart deformities, the majority do not survive beyond the first year. Figures obtained from hospital records show that 60 percent of all mongoloids born alive do not survive beyond 10 years of age. The distinguished human geneticist Lionel S. Penrose places the life expectancy of mongoloids at 12 years.

Mongoloid children have a strange assortment of other defects. The neck is short and broad, the skin is rosy but rough and dry, the teeth are abnormally shaped and irregularly aligned, and the gonads and genitalia are underdeveloped. The males surviving to reproductive age are sterile; there is no known case of a mongoloid father having children. Mongoloid

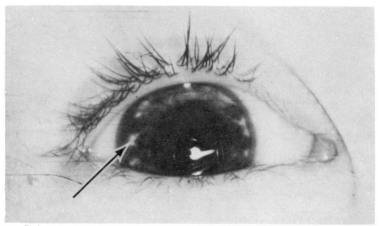

FIG. 5-4 CLOUDLIKE, WHITISH SPOTTING of the iris of the eye, characteristically found at birth in mongoloid infants. (Courtesy of Dr. Norman Woody, Tulane University School of Medicine.)

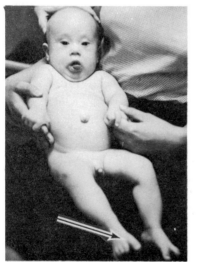
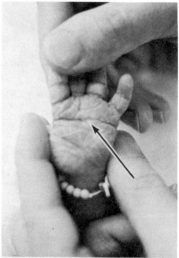

FIG. 5-5 MONGOLOID INFANT showing the short, incurving fifth finger; the wide gap between the first and second toes; and the strong crease in the palm, the so-called "simian line." (From C. B. Jacobson, "Cytogenetic techniques and their clinical uses," in *Genetics in Medical Practice,* edited by M. Bartalos, J.B. Lippincott Company, Philadelphia, 1965.)

females have fared better; 13 females with offspring have been recorded. In essence, the vast majority never reproduce. Afflicted children thus usually come from normal parents.

A peculiar feature of mongoloid infants is the speckled appearance of the iris of the eye. Numerous and distinct whitish spots, technically referred to as "Brushfield's spots," named for the British doctor Thomas Brushfield (1858–1937), are concentrically arranged on the surface of the iris (FIG. 5–4). Speckling has been found in approximately 90 percent of afflicted individuals at birth and accordingly is of particular value for purposes of diagnosis. Similar spots may be found in normal newborn infants, but they are less numerous and less distinct.

Many unusual features of mongoloids' hands have been reported. Typically broad and stumpy, the hands are from 10 to 30 percent shorter than normal hands. In particular, the fifth, or "little" finger is abnormally small and incurved (FIG. 5–5). The dermatoglyphic, or ridge, patterns of the fingers, palms, and soles are grossly abnormal. On the finger tips, the dermal ridges are arranged primarily in loops; normal patterns such as whorls and arches are greatly reduced in number. The palm of the hand has a prominent single transverse fold or crease, the so-called "simian line." The feet, often short and clumsy, have a characteristic well-marked gap between the first and second toe (FIG. 5–5).

Incidence and Cause

MEDICAL SCIENTISTS had speculated for many decades on the possible causes of mongolism. It did not escape their attention that mongoloids were born more often to older women. The incidence of mongolism rises markedly with maternal age (FIG. 5–6). The incidence of mongoloid births is one per 1,500 among women under 30, one per 750 at maternal ages 30-34, one per 600 at ages 35-39, and one per 300 among mothers at ages 40-45. Among women over 45, one in 30 infants may be expected to be mongoloid! About 7,000 mongoloids are born each year in the United States, and the great majority are born to mothers over 35 years of age. The age of the father appears to be of little or no significance.

Medical opinion erred grievously for a long time in recognizing the true cause of mongolism. At one time or another, syphilis, tuberculosis, psychic shock, thyroid deficiency, and even alcoholism were incriminated as causes of mongolism. However, by the 1930's, genetic influences were acknowledged. The idea that genetic factors were important came from studies of mongolism among monozygotic (identical) and dizygotic (fraternal) twins. In identical twins, both members are invariably mongoloid. Among fraternal twins, if one is affected, the other is rarely mongoloid, even though both share the same maternal environment. Moreover, in any family, the parents are almost always normal, and it is unusual for more than one child to be affected. These considerations pointed to some alteration in the genetic material of the parents, transmissible to the child.

In 1959, the young pediatrician Jérôme Lejeune and his colleagues, Marthe Gauthier and Raymond Turpin, at the University of Paris, studied the chromosomes of cells taken from the skin of mongoloid idiots. They employed the newly discovered technique of culturing the skin cells and preparing the cells for chromosome analysis. It came as a curious surprise when Lejeune and his collaborators found that the cells of mongol chil-

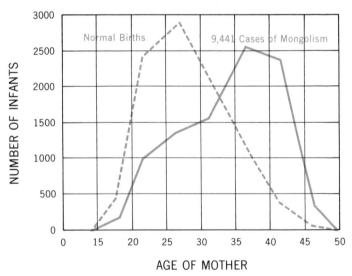

FIG. 5–6 GRAPHIC REPRESENTATION of the increased incidence of Down's syndrome (mongolism) with advancing age of the mother. (Based on data by Dr. L. S. Penrose, Harperbury Hospital, Hertfordshire, England.)

dren do not contain the normal chromosome number of 46, but rather 47. The additional chromosome was one of the very small chromosomes, but this slight excess of genetic material was sufficient to disrupt the normal developmental processes.

We have seen that several different parts of the body are affected in mongoloid children. An extra chromosome means that numerous genes are represented three times rather than twice. Since a given chromosome carries a variety of genes with different functions, an additional complement of the various genes would be expected to disturb several different bodily processes. The strange assortment of defects seen in mongoloid children is thus explicable.

Aged Eggs

THERE IS STRONG EVIDENCE that the extra chromosome of the mongoloid infant is acquired during the production of the egg of the mother. A mishap occurs in the behavior of the chromo-

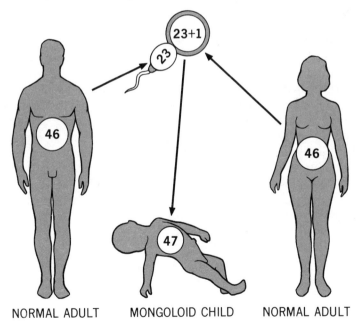

NORMAL ADULT   MONGOLOID CHILD   NORMAL ADULT

FIG. 5–7 THE TRUE CAUSE of mongolism. Mongoloid children do not have the normal chromosome number of 46, but rather 47. The extra chromosome of the mongoloid infant is acquired during the production of the egg of the mother.

somes during the formation of the egg from which the child develops. The exact mechanism of such a "mistake" will be discussed in the next chapter. For the moment, the essential consideration is that the mongoloid child arises when a defective egg with 24 chromosomes is fertilized by a normal sperm with 23 chromosomes (FIG. 5-7).

All the eggs that a woman produces during her reproductive life are present from the moment of birth. In fact, her eggs are nested in her ovaries months before she is born. At birth, the ovaries contain at least 500,000 cells known as oocytes—that is, immature or prospective egg cells. The egg of a 20-year-old woman matures from an oocyte that has "rested" for 20 years, whereas the egg of a 40-year-old woman has been dormant for 40 years. The maturation of eggs from the oocytes is apparently impaired with advancing age. In other words, there is a progressive decline of the number of eggs that mature perfectly as the woman ages. By the age of 50, the production of functional eggs is typically no longer possible.

We began this chapter by discussing Witschi's study which showed that overripeness of the eggs of frogs leads to all sorts of anomalies. There is now every reason to believe that the eggs of the human female are subject to the same hazards. Indeed, Dr. James German, a geneticist at Cornell University, suggested in 1968 that the higher risk of mongolism in babies born to older women may be related to the decreasing frequency of sexual intercourse in marriages of long standing. Since sexual relations tend to become less frequent or sporadic after the early years of marriage, the chances are greater in older women that sperm may not be present to fertilize the egg as soon as it is released from the ovary. Dr. German contends that infrequent sexual relations and the consequent danger of delayed fertilization are important factors governing the incidence of mongoloid births.

Young Mothers of Mongoloids

THAT THE EGGS SUFFER degenerative changes with the woman's advancing age explains the high incidence of mongolism in older women, but leaves unexplained the occasional birth of a mongoloid child to a *mother in her early twenties*.

This particular problem attracted the attention of a team of British investigators, Drs. P. E. Polani, J. H. Briggs, C. E. Ford, C. M. Clarke, and J. M. Berg. They analyzed the chromosomes in the bone marrow cells of a mongoloid girl born to a mother only 21 years old. They found 46 chromosomes in the child instead of the expected 47. However, detailed examination of the chromosomes revealed that one of the chromosomes had an unusual configuration. It appeared to consist of two chromosomes fused together. The interpretation advanced was that the mongoloid child had inherited an extra chromosome but that this extra chromosome had become integrally joined to another chromosome. Stated another way, one chromosome was in fact represented three times, but the third was almost concealed on another chromosome. An understanding of this odd phenomenon requires specific knowledge of the kinds of chromosomes in humans, the subject of the next chapter.

Chapter 6

The Human Chromosome Complement

IN THE 1920's, Dr. Theophilus S. Painter (1889–1969), the eminent geneticist at the University of Texas, made a valiant attempt to count the chromosomes in cells obtained from the testes of a human subject. Using techniques that are crude and laborious by modern standards, he estimated that the number of chromosomes in the body cells of man is 48 (FIG. 6–1). Confidence in this number developed to a point where it was believed to represent one of the unequivocal facts about the human species.

With the perfection of techniques in the 1950's which allowed growth of human cells *in vitro* (outside of the body), new avenues of approaches to the study of human cells were realized. In 1956, Drs. J. H. Tjio and Albert Levan, of the Institute of Genetics at Lund in Sweden, electrified the biological world with the announcement that the cells of the lungs of a human fetus, grown in laboratory cultures, were found to possess only 46 chromosomes. The pictures of the chromosomes which they presented were of a degree of clarity previously

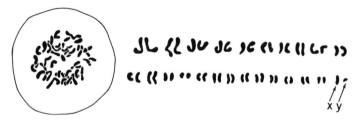

FIG. 6–1 CHROMOSOMES of a human male, arranged in 24 pairs by Dr. T. S. Painter in 1923. Modern preparations of human cells reveal, beyond any reasonable doubt, that man possesses 23 pairs of chromosomes, not 24 pairs (see FIG. 6–4).

unequaled for human cells. Their unexpected finding was soon confirmed by a host of other investigators. The correct number of chromosomes in man is not 48, as had been believed for decades, but 46.

The Division of Cells

ONE CAN SCARCELY INTERPRET satisfactorily a picture of human chromosomes without an understanding of the process by which cells divide. The formation of new cells in the body is a continual process, although certain cells divide more often than others, and some not at all. Cells in the skin, intestine, and blood-forming tissues divide often to replace those that are continually being worn out. Kidney and liver cells are renewed less often, and certain highly specialized cells, such as nerve cells, are not replaced when damaged.

The nucleus of a cell ordinarily has a netted appearance (FIG. 6-2). Early investigators found that the fine network of the material in the nucleus stains deeply with certain dyes, such as the purple coloring matter known as hematoxylin. Because of its affinity for dyes, the substance making up the net was termed "chromatin," from *chroma,* Greek for color. The chromatin net is actually a tangled mass of thin threads, the chromosomes. The chromosomes are packed like a ball of yarn and, hence, are not individually recognizable. A cell at this stage is described as "resting." This is a misnomer, as the "resting" cell is actually involved in intense activity to maintain the life of the cell. The cell at this time is more properly said to be in the interphase stage.

When a cell begins to divide, the chromosomes become discernible as separate threadlike strands. This early stage of division is known as the prophase. In our simple illustrative example (FIG. 6-2), only four chromosomes are represented. As the chromosomes become shorter and thicker, it becomes apparent that each chromosome consists of two daughter strands. The longitudinal doubling of the chromosomes had actually occurred during the resting stage. Each longitudinal half of a chromosome is termed a chromatid. The two daughter chromatids are joined only at a region known as the centromere.

By the time the chromosomes are distinguishable as longitu-

MITOSIS

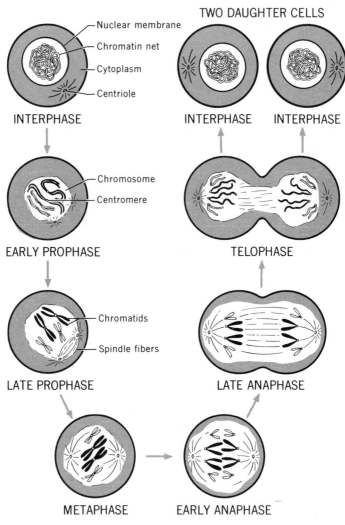

FIG. 6–2 MITOSIS, the process by which body cells divide, is illustrated for a cell with four chromosomes. The two daughter cells each have four chromosomes, the same number as the original cell.

dinally doubled, rodlike structures, other changes have taken place. The delicate membrane which surrounds the nucleus has disappeared. Two small bodies lying outside the nucleus, known as centrioles, migrate to opposite poles of the cell and give rise to a series of fine lines, the spindle fibers. The chromosomes now collect in the center of the spindle, and are attached to the spindle fibers by their centromeres with their arms extending outward. This stage is referred to as the metaphase. It is at this time that the chromosomes are maximally contracted and most conspicuous microscopically.

The centromere of each chromosome then divides, and the spindle fibers pull the chromatids, now daughter chromosomes, to the opposite poles of the cell (the "anaphase" stage). At the same moment, the cell pinches in two. Around each cluster of daughter chromosomes, a new nuclear membrane forms. The protoplasm of the cell completes its separation into two new, or daughter, cells during the teleophase stage. The spindle fibers vanish, the chromosomes lose their distinct outlines, and the two new cells assume the appearance of resting cells.

This process by which new cells in the body arise from pre-existing cells was termed "mitosis" by the German anatomist Walther Flemming (1843–1905) in 1882. The process ensures that the two daughter cells receive identical copies of the chromosome complement of the parent cell. The process also permits us to interpret the configurations seen in a preparation of human chromosomes.

Normal Human Chromosome Complement

UNTIL VERY RECENTLY the study of human chromosomes had been hampered by technical difficulties. As we have seen, the chromosomes are most readily visible during the metaphase state, when the chromosomes are short and thick. This is but a brief period in the division of the cell. Moreover, in ordinary microscopic preparations of dividing cells, such as those of Painter's study (FIG. 6-1), the numerous human chromosomes appear hopelessly crowded.

The last 15 years have witnessed an explosive surge of new techniques. The first major advance was the perfection of procedures for culturing cells *in vitro*. The second innovation was the application to human cell cultures of colchicine, a chemical substance obtained from the roots of the autumn crocus plant. The addition of colchicine to cultures of human cells provided large numbers of dividing cells in metaphase, due to the unique action of colchicine in arresting cell division permanently at the metaphase stage.

There remained, however, the problem of spreading apart the clustered metaphase chromosomes. Human cells are normally grown in a balanced saline medium, one that contains concentrations of salts that approximate the salt content of blood. In 1952, Dr. T. C. Hsu of the University of Texas introduced an unbalanced, or hypotonic, salt solution to his preparation of dividing cells. The hypotonic solution (of low salt concentration) forced the cells to absorb water and swell. In

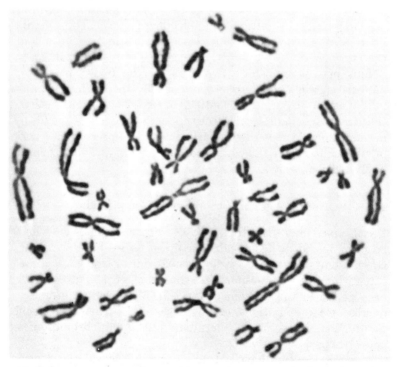

FIG. 6–3 SPREAD-OUT SET of normal human chromosomes in the nucleus of a blood cell of a male. Each chromosome consists of two strands joined at the centromere. (Prepared by Elizabeth M. Earley, Tulane University.)

dramatic fashion, the metaphase chromosomes scattered, spreading out individually over a large area.

It remained for Drs. Tjio and Levan of Sweden in 1956 to employ the new techniques to discover that man had 46 chromosomes. But the technical advances did not stop there. From the research laboratory of Dr. Peter Nowell of the University of Pennsylvania School of Medicine there emerged another important finding. He observed that phytohemagglutinin, a substance extracted from red kidney beans, could stimulate the human white blood cells (leucocytes) to divide in the culture medium. This made possible the preparation of metaphase chromosomes from peripheral (circulating) blood, which of course can be obtained much more readily from the body than internal solid tissues.

A chromosome spread prepared from a culture of blood cells of a human male is shown in FIGURE 6–3. As expected from our knowledge of metaphase chromosomes, each chromosome is longitudinally doubled, and the two strands (or chromatids) are tied together by a centromere. You will recall also that the chromosomes occur in pairs, one member of each chromosome coming from the mother and the other from the father. Thus, each chromosome has a partner, the two constituting a pair of like, or "homologous," chromosomes.

The chromosomes can be systematically arranged in a sequence known as a karyotype (FIG. 6–4). In preparing the karyotype, the chromosomes are paired and classified into groups according to size and position of the centromere. A centromere situated in the middle divides the chromosome into two arms of equal length. When the centromere is located away from the midline, one arm appears longer than the other. In some chromosomes, the centromere is nearly terminal in position, imparting a wishbone appearance to the chromosome.

There are 22 matching pairs of chromosomes which are called *autosomes.* The autosome pairs are numbered 1 to 22 in descending order of length, and further classified into seven groups, designated by capital letters, A through G. In addition, there are two *sex chromosomes,* which are unnumbered. As seen in FIGURE 6–4, the male has one X chromosome and one unequal-sized Y chromosome. The female has two X chromosomes of equal size and no Y chromosome. Thus, the 46 hu-

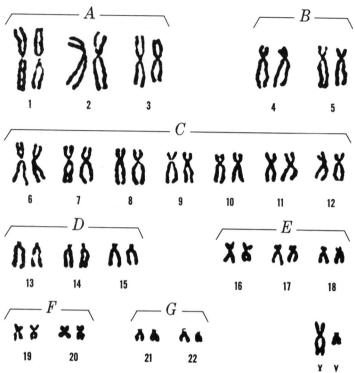

FIG. 6–4 THE 23 PAIRS of chromosomes of a normal male arranged from the chromosomes of the cell shown in FIG. 6–3. (Prepared by Elizabeth M. Earley, Tulane University.)

man chromosomes comprise 22 pairs of autosomes plus the sex chromosome pair, XX in normal females and XY in normal males. The 46 chromosomes constitute the diploid set (Greek, *diploos,* meaning double). The haploid set *(haploos,* single), found in sperm and egg cells, consists of 22 autosomes plus one of the sex chromosomes, or a total of 23.

FIGURE 6–4 shows clearly that the male Y is one of the smallest chromosomes, and considerably smaller than the X. It has been estimated that the female has four percent more genetic material in each of her cells than does the male. This rather extraordinary situation will merit our attention in a subsequent chapter.

Trisomy 21 and Meiosis

WE MAY NOW RETURN to the discovery by Dr. Lejeune and his associates of an extra chromosome in the cells of mongoloid children (see Chapter 5). The additional chromosome turns out to be one of the small chromosomes (No. 21) in Group G. Mongoloid children are said to display trisomy (three rather than two) of chromosome 21, or, simply, trisomy 21. This condition is made possible by a mishap in the behavior of the chromosomes during the formation of the egg from which the child developed. How the peculiar accident might arise requires an understanding of the chromosomal events during the production of the gametes.

The gametes are derived from specialized cells—sperm from spermatogonia in the testes of the male and eggs from oogonia in the ovary of the female (FIG. 6–5). These specialized cells, like other body cells, contain 46 chromosomes. Obviously some mechanism must exist whereby the number of chromosomes is reduced in half in each of the gametes. This mechanism is termed *meiosis.*

Two meiotic divisions are involved in the formation of the gametes (FIG. 6–5). In the first meiotic division, each chromosome becomes longitudinally doubled as in mitosis, but the centromeres do not divide nor do the daughter chromatids separate from each other. Rather, each chromosome is attracted to, and pairs lengthwise with, its homologous chromosome. During the first meiotic division, the homologous chromosomes migrate to opposite poles of the spindle, resulting in two daughter cells, each with half the original number of chromosomes. The second meiotic division involves, like mitosis, the division of the centromere and the separation of the chromatids of each chromosome into the daughter cells. The end product consists of gametes that have half the chromosome number of the body cells, or the haploid number.

Each spermatogonial cell in the testes of the male produces four sperm cells. The process of meiosis is essentially the same in the female, except that the division of the cytoplasm is unequal (FIG. 6–5). In the first division of the oocyte (more properly, the primary oocyte), one of the two cells, the first polar body, receives very little cytoplasm, while the other, the secon-

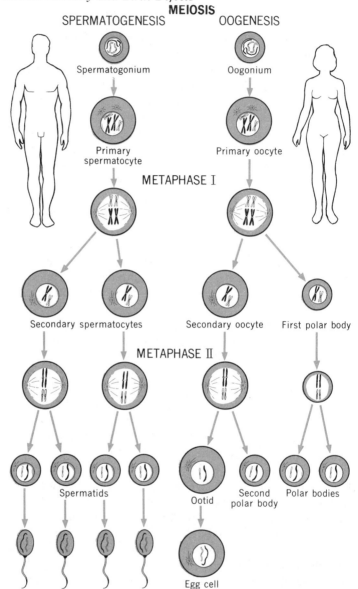

FIG. 6-5 MEIOSIS, the process by which the gametes, sperm and egg, come to possess only half the full number of chromosomes. In this illustrative example, the number of chromosomes is reduced from four in the original cells to two in the gametes.

dary oocyte, receives a massive amount. At the second meiotic division, the secondary oocyte divides into an egg cell with most of the cytoplasm and another polar body (the second polar body) with a scant amount of cytoplasm. The first polar body may undergo a mitotic division simultaneously (FIG. 6–5). All polar bodies disintegrate, leaving the mature egg or ovum. The egg has 23 chromosomes, including one X chromosome.

The process of meiosis is complex, and subject to error. It does not always proceed normally. Occasional accidents do occur that affect the normal functioning of the spindle fibers and impede the proper migration of one or more chromosomes.

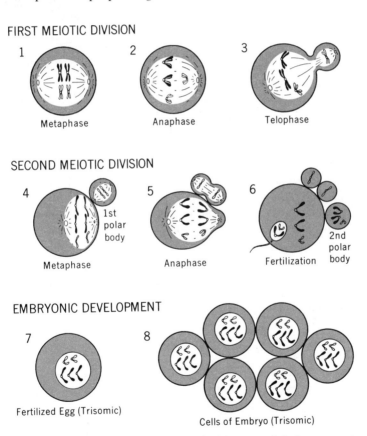

FIRST MEIOTIC DIVISION

1 Metaphase   2 Anaphase   3 Telophase

SECOND MEIOTIC DIVISION

4 Metaphase   1st polar body   5 Anaphase   6 Fertilization   2nd polar body

EMBRYONIC DEVELOPMENT

7 Fertilized Egg (Trisomic)   8 Cells of Embryo (Trisomic)

FIG. 6–6 NONDISJUNCTION DURING MEIOSIS produces an egg cell that possesses two of a given chromosome rather than the usual one. Such an egg cell, when fertilized by a normal sperm, would give rise to a defective trisomic individual.

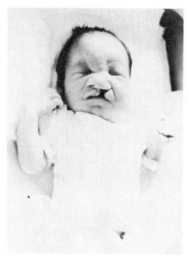 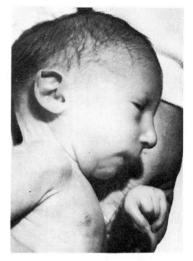

FIG. 6–7 DEFORMED INFANTS possessing an extra group D chromosome *(left)* and an extra group E chromosome *(right)*, respectively. (From C. B. Jacobson, "Cytogenetic techniques and their clinical uses," *Genetics in Medical Practice*, edited by M. Bartalos, J. B. Lippincott Company, Philadelphia, 1965.)

During the first meiotic division, it may happen that a given pair of chromosomes fail to separate from each other (FIG. 6–6). This failure of separation, known as *nondisjunction*, results in an egg cell containing both members of a given pair of chromosomes. The nondisjunction of the 21st pair of chromosomes, for example, would result in an egg cell that possessed two 21st chromosomes rather than the usual one. Such an egg cell, when fertilized by a normal sperm, would give rise to an individual that is trisomic for the 21st chromosome, or a mongoloid idiot.

Trisomy of other Autosomes

THEORETICALLY ANY ONE of the chromosomes may occur in the trisomic state. Two syndromes of severe deformities have been traced to an extra group D chromosome and to an extra group E chromosome, respectively (FIG. 6–7). Among newborns, about one in 1,000 have a group D chromosome in triplicate; about one in 1,500 are trisomic for one of the E chromosomes (typically No. 18). Both trisomic conditions, resulting in an abnormal count of 47 chromosomes, are usually fatal within the first year of life.

Common anomalies in trisomy D include cleft palate (often with harelip), sloping forehead with relatively small braincase, defective eye development, and polydactyly. Developmental disorders of the heart and kidney contribute to an early death of the infant. Common clinical features of trisomy E infants are a recessed chin, malformed ears, spasticity due to a defective nervous system, and peculiarly pliable fingers (FIG. 6–7).

Since many more genes are carried in the larger chromosomes, trisomies involving the large chromosomes (such as those of the A and B groups) are likely to have lethal consequences. Recent studies indicate that 40 percent of all embryos which are aborted during the first three months of pregnancy have some sort of chromosomal error. Some of the spontaneous abortions are due to trisomies of the medium-sized and large-sized autosomes.

Translocation Errors

NOT ALL CHROMOSOMAL ERRORS involve nondisjunction of a pair of chromosomes. Another chromosomal aberration is *translocation*. This occurs when two chromosomes break and then rejoin in the wrong combination (FIG. 6–8). We alluded to this phenomenon in our earlier discussion (Chapter 5) of Ford's observation of a mongoloid child born to a 21-year-old mother. In this particular case, the translocation occurred in the mother's cells between a normal chromosome No. 15 and a

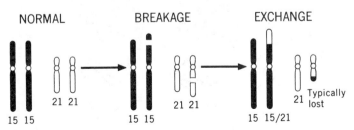

FIG. 6–8 PHENOMENON OF TRANSLOCATION produces a single large chromosome (designated 15/21) and a small fragment which is usually lost without affecting the person adversely.

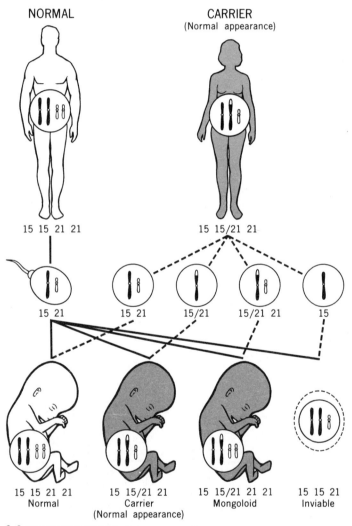

FIG. 6-9 TRANSLOCATION-TYPE MONGOLISM carries a great risk of producing additional mongoloid children. One viable offspring in three will be mongoloid. Of the other two viable offspring, one will be a carrier of mongolism for future generations.

normal chromosome No. 21. As seen in FIGURE 6–8, unequal pieces of chromosomes were exchanged, resulting in a single large chromosome that incorporates the greater part of both chromosomes 15 and 21. This newly formed large chromosome is designated as the 15/21 translocation chromosome. The small fragment containing relatively few genes is lost, but this is without consequence. The consequences, however, of the mother bearing the 15/21 chromosome are vast for her children.

FIGURE 6–9 shows a woman carrying the 15/21 translocation chromosome. She is normal in appearance! When she produces eggs, some will contain two No. 21 chromosomes (one of them fused to chromosome 15) and others will have none. Specifically, she will produce four kinds of eggs (FIG. 6–9), which, when fertilized by normal sperm, would result in four possible outcomes: (1) a completely normal child with an entirely normal chromosome set; (2) a normal child that has the 15/21 translocation chromosome like the mother, and has the potential to inflict her children with translocation-type mongolism; (3) a mongoloid child with three No. 21 chromosomes, one of which is fused to chromosome 15; and (4) an embryo that lacks completely one of the pairs of chromosome 21 and dies before term.

Unlike mongolism associated with advancing maternal age (nondisjunction trisomy 21), translocation-type mongolism "runs" in families. In other words, there is a frequent occurrence of mongoloid births. As we have seen, the risk of a mongoloid child among those developing to term is one chance in three. If the child is not mongoloid, there is one chance in two that the child will be a carrier of translocation-type mongolism. This contrasts sharply with nondisjunction trisomy, where the risk of giving birth to an affected child is about one in 600.

The 15/21 translocation event is not necessarily confined to the mother. The consequences to the child are the same if the translocation occurred in the father. Cases are known in which the father has been implicated as the carrier. And, like sheltered recessive genes, the 15/21 translocated chromosome can be transmitted through several generations without detection, since the probability of a mongoloid birth would be one-third, the remaining offspring being apparently normal.

Deletion of Genetic Material

SOMETIMES A PIECE OF CHROMOSOME breaks off, resulting in a *deletion* of genetic material. The effects of the loss of a portion of a chromosome depend on the particular genes lost. A major deletion, with the loss of many genes, is incompatible with life.

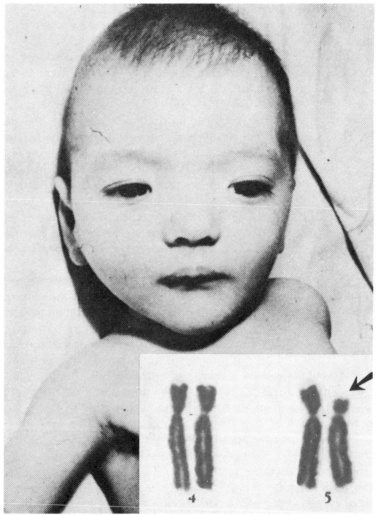

FIG. 6-10 MOONLIKE FACE of infant suffering from the loss of a portion of the No. 5 chromosome. (Courtesy of Dr. Jérôme Lejeune, Université de Paris, France.)

Dr. Jérôme Lejeune and his colleagues at the University of Paris described in 1963 the peculiar effects in an infant of the loss of one of a portion of the No. 5 chromosome (group B). Affected infants have a rounded, moonlike face and utter feeble, plaintive cries described as similar to the mewing of a cat (FIG. 6–10). In fact, the disorder has been named the *"cri du chat"* ("cat cry") syndrome. Such unfortunate infants remain mentally and physically retarded. Although originally thought to be exceedingly rare, at least 70 cases of the cri du chat disorder have been reported since the initial discovery.

The Philadelphia Chromosome and Leukemia

LEUKEMIA IS A cancerous malignancy arising in the blood-forming tissues. Like cancer in general, leukemia is a clinically heterogeneous entity, appearing in many forms. In 1960, Drs. Peter Nowell and D. A. Hungerford noted the presence of an exceptionally minute chromosome in dividing cells from the bone marrow of patients with chronic myeloid leukemia. This particular form of leukemia is characterized by abnormal numbers of immature granulocytes (one of the white blood cells) in bone marrow and blood. The unusually small chromosome, evidently with a piece missing, proved to be one of the 21st pair. The patient with chronic myeloid leukemia thus has 46 chromosomes, but chromosome No. 21 is marred by a deletion. Because the finding was made in Philadelphia, the abnormal chromosome has been called the Philadelphia chromosome.

The association between leukemia and the chromosome aberration suggests that the hereditary material of the 21st chromosome is concerned with the maturation of blood cells. This supposition is given added weight by the finding that the incidence of leukemia in mongoloid individuals is nearly six times that of normal persons. It will be recalled that mongolism is a disorder involving the 21st chromosome.

These observations strongly indicate a close relationship between a chromosomal error and cancer. However, it may be that the chromosomal deletion does not cause the abnormal growth, but is rather the consequence of malignancy.

Drugs and Chromosomes

IT NOW APPEARS that several familiar drugs may cause breaks or other abnormalities in the chromosomes. Abnormally high numbers of broken chromosomes have been found in cultures of human blood cells to which have been added chloropromazine (a popular tranquilizer), or diphenhydramine (a major antihistamine), or LSD (the euphoric hallucinogen). A cause-and-effect relationship between LSD (lysergic acid diethylamide) and abnormalities in the infants of pregnant mothers who took LSD has not been unequivocally established. But circumstantial evidence is strong. The drug became a prime suspect when some of the infants of mothers who had taken LSD during pregnancy had a damaged chromosome resembling the aforementioned Philadelphia chromosome, associated with chronic myeloid leukemia. This form of cancer is rare, and its occurrence in several infants suggests more than a coincidence. Evidently, LSD should not be taken except for sound medical reasons—but there does *not* seem to exist a single sound reason.

Chapter 7

Sex Chromosomes and Abnormalities

IN THE FALL OF 1967, Ewa Klobukowska, Polish co-holder of the woman's 100-meter dash record (11.1 seconds), was disqualified from European Cup competition at Kiev. Russian and Hungarian doctors had examined her chromosomes and held that she was more man than woman. The curt medical announcement was that Ewa has "one chromosome too many."

Ewa's case has stirred up confusion and resentment. Her fiancé, a student at Warsaw's Economics College which she also attends, remains astonished at the suggestion that Ewa may not be all female. The controversy flared in the spring of 1968, when Ewa, who also holds an Olympic gold medal, was ordered stripped of her records and medals because she had failed the "sex test" in 1967. That same spring, the International Olympic Committee announced that all woman athletes would be tested for sex prior to the Olympic games to "discourage countries from entering doubtful contestants."

A normal female differs from the normal male in carrying two X chromosomes; the male is XY. Sex is determined at the moment of conception. A female arises from the union of an X-bearing egg with an X-bearing sperm, whereas a male results from the X-bearing egg being fertilized by a Y-bearing sperm (FIG. 7–1). It is the Y chromosome that establishes maleness.

A few individuals do suffer from various kinds of errors in their sex chromosomes. A relatively common case of "one chromosome too many" is an XXY combination, but this is accompanied by external male genitalia (although underdeveloped) and poor physical development, certainly not at all characteristic of athletes. Thus, Ewa Klobukowska's problem, if any, still remains unclear to medical scientists.

Klinefelter's Syndrome

A SEX ANOMALY in males that occurs as high as one in 800 births is Klinefelter's syndrome, named after Harry F. Klinefelter, an American physician who first described it in 1942. Although individuals with this syndrome are male in general

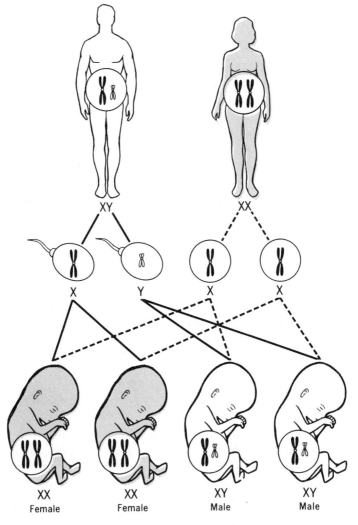

FIG. 7-1 NORMAL INHERITANCE PATTERN of sex, in which the chance of producing a girl (XX) or a boy (XY) is equal (one-half chance in each case).

appearance, their testes are underdeveloped and their breasts are enlarged (FIG. 7-2). Their limbs are longer than average and body hair is sparse. Most patients are sterile and many are mentally defective.

In 1959, Patricia A. Jacobs and J. A. Strong at an Edinburgh

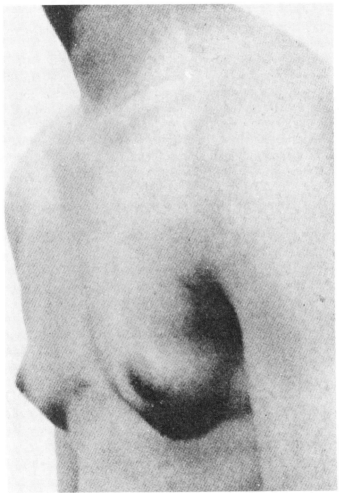

FIG. 7-2 KLINEFELTER'S SYNDROME occurs in males whose Y chromosome is accompanied by two X chromosomes instead of one. One symptom is enlarged breasts. (From H. F. Klinefelter, E. C. Reifenstein, and F. Albright, *Journal of Clinical Endocrinology* 2: 615, 1942. (With permission of the J. B. Lippincott Company, Philadelphia.)

hospital discovered that the cells of males with Klinefelter's syndrome have 47 chromosomes instead of 46. A normal Y is present, but the X chromosome is represented twice. Thus, these sterile males possess an XXY sex-chromosome constitution. In subsequent years, males with XXXY (triplo-X), XXXXY (tetra-X), and XXXXXY (penta-X) constitutions were observed. Despite numerous X chromosomes, the presence of the Y chromosome enables the patient to have masculine characteristics.

As in mongolism, affected males are born more often to older women. The extra X chromosome arises as a consequence of nondisjunction of the sex chromosomes during the formation of eggs by the mother. The mother produces either an XX egg or an egg devoid of sex chromosomes (FIG. 7-3). In some cases, it is suspected that the father produces an abnormal XY sperm through nondisjunction. Thus, either the fertilization of an XX egg by a normal Y sperm or the union of a normal X egg and an XY sperm would result in Klinefelter's syndrome.

Many geneticists were dismayed when it turned out that an XXY individual is a sterile male. In the fruit fly, long the favorite subject of study by geneticists, an XXY individual is a normal, fertile female!

Turner's Syndrome

THROUGH NONDISJUNCTION, eggs can be produced which have no X chromosome at all. When such an egg is fertilized by an X-bearing sperm, the offspring will be XO, "O" signifying the absence of a sex chromosome (FIG. 7-3). Such an individual, possessing only one sex chromosome (the X), has a total of 45 chromosomes. In 1959, Dr. C. E. Ford and his co-workers in England detected the XO constitution in women suffering from Turner's syndrome, an anomaly first noticed in 1938 by Dr. Henry H. Turner of the University of Oklahoma School of Medicine. Women with Turner's syndrome have rudimentary ovaries, if any at all, and undeveloped breasts. Anatomically and psychologically they are females, although unable to menstruate or ovulate. Instead of normal ovaries, only ridges of whitish tissue occur, a finding which has caused the term "streak gonads" to be applied. In addition, many authors use the term "gonadal dysgenesis" in place of Turner's syndrome.

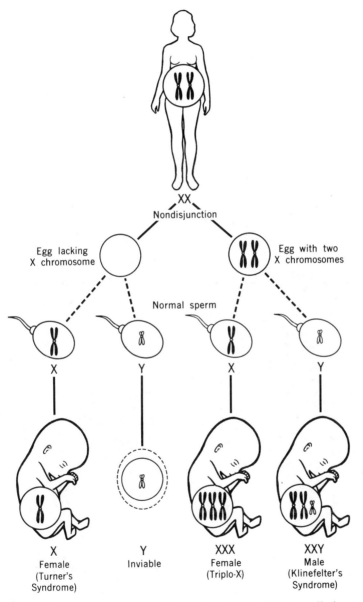

FIG. 7-3 NONDISJUNCTION can result in an egg cell containing two X chromosomes rather than one, and an egg cell containing no X chromosomes ("O"). Only defective offspring can arise from such eggs.

Affected women are also unusually short, have a peculiar webbing of the skin of the neck (FIG. 7-4), and are of subnormal intelligence.

The XO woman is not a case of sex reversal, since testes and other male components are absent. Rather, she is an undeveloped female who would have developed as a normal female had she not been denied the other X chromosome. Curiously, XO individuals in humans are sterile females, whereas XO fruit flies are sterile males. Nondisjunction of the sex chromosomes may occur during the formation of the egg or sperm. In the majority of cases, the X is probably of maternal origin.

It may also happen that an X chromosome is lost during an early cell division of the embryo. In this event, the infant is a genetic mosaic, with some cells XO and others XX. That this possibility may actually occur is indicated by the findings in 1961 of Dr. Raymond Turpin and his colleagues in France. A

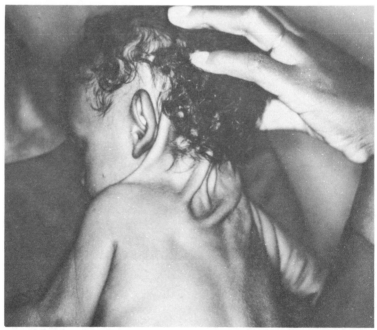

FIG. 7-4 TURNER'S SYNDROME is found in females with only one X chromosome. A characteristic feature is the "webbing" of the neck. (Courtesy of Dr. Norman Woody, Tulane University School of Medicine.)

pair of monozygotic (identical) twins was analyzed in which one member was male with an XY constitution and the other a sterile female with an XO constitution. Clearly, the XO condition originated by the loss of one of the sex chromosomes when the single fertilized egg divided into two.

The incidence of Turner's syndrome is surprisingly low, one in 3,500 births, in comparison to the incidence of Klinefelter's syndrome (one in 800 births). The most probable explanation is that many fetuses afflicted with Turner's syndrome die before term.

Not all instances of "streak gonads" are associated with the XO constitution. Rare cases are known in which the females have rudimentary "streak" ovaries and lack secondary sexual characteristics. They are, however, normal in stature and do not display the conspicuous "short necks" of women suffering from Turner's syndrome. This condition is known as "pure" gonadal dysgenesis. Ironically, many of these sterile females have a male chromosome complement, 46 chromosomes including the XY. The condition appears to be due to a defective gene or genes, which suppresses in some way the male-determining function of the Y chromosome.

The Triplo-X Female

GENTICISTS WORKING WITH fruit flies designated females with three X chromosomes as "super-females." This label is inappropriate for the human females with three X's, a condition which predisposes to mental retardation and infertility. However, some triplo-X females have no apparent physical abnormalities and most are fertile.

Most children born to triplo-X females have been either normal males or normal females. This is surprising, since the triplo-X mother would be expected to produce two kinds of eggs (XX-bearing and X-bearing), and, accordingly, half of her sons would be XXY (Klinefelter's syndrome) and half of her daughters would have the triplo-X condition. It might well be that XX eggs are inviable; that is, only X-bearing eggs are functional.

From FIGURE 7–3, it is seen that one other type of offspring is theoretically possible. This is the YO zygote, resulting from the union of an egg lacking an X-chromosome with a Y-bearing sperm. The YO constitution apparently is incompatible with life; no such individual has been found.

Sex Determination

FOR MANY YEARS, the genetic sex-determining mechanism in the fruit fly (Drosophila) has served as a model for other organisms, including man. In Drosophila, sex is governed largely by the X chromosome—an XXY fly is a fertile female and an XO fly is a sterile male. The Y chromosome is essentially inert in relation to sex determination, although necessary for male fertility.

In humans, it is clear that the Y chromosome, far from having a passive role in sex determination, contains potent male-determining genes. An individual who carries a Y chromosome is a male, even if he has one, two, or three X chromosomes associated with the Y. An individual lacking the Y chromosome is a female, whether she be XO, XX, or XXX.

The statement that maleness in humans is a function of the Y chromosome requires some qualification. Most true hermaphrodites—individuals in which both ovarian and testicular tissues are present—have 46 chromosomes with an XX constitution. None of the hermaphrodites are fertile, although egg and sperm may be formed. The presence of testicular tissue in hermaphrodites tends to negate the view that the Y chromosome is necessary for the formation of a testis. However, a few hermaphrodites have been found to be "mosaics," that is, containing cells of two kinds, XX and XY. The mosaic state would make possible the development of both testicular and ovarian tissue. The possibility thus remains that all hermaphrodites with an apparent XX constitution originate as XX/XY mosaics, but the XY cells are either lost or undetected.

The XYY Male

THE EVIDENCE INDICATES that the Y chromosome is strongly male-determining. Conceivably an extra Y chromosome might cause overaggressiveness through an overproduction of male hormones. There are actual indications that men of XYY constitutions are prone to violence and antisocial behavior.

The occurrence of an XYY chromosome abnormality was first reported in 1962 by Dr. T. S. Hauschka and his co-workers at the Roswell Park Memorial Institute in Buffalo, New York. A possible link between the abnormal karyotype and aberrant behavior was first suggested in 1965 when the XYY complement was detected in nearly four percent of the inmates at a maximum-security prison in Lanarkshire, Scotland. Subsequent surveys in Britain and North America lent support to the possibility that the additional Y chromosome increases predisposition to criminality. The afflicted males are usually taller than average (more than 6 feet tall), tend to have barely normal IQ's, and suffer persistent acne. The XYY constitution is suspected to occur in one in 300 males.

Thus far, geneticists have more questions than answers about the XYY male. A number of XYY males do not have the physical or behavioral characteristics assumed to be associated with the extra Y chromosome. It is premature to con-

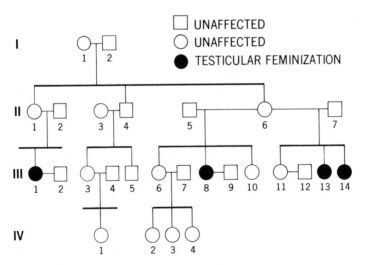

FIG. 7-5 PEDIGREE OF TESTICULAR FEMINIZATION. Affected persons are females but have testes and an XY constitution. The transmission of the defective condition is from mother to daughter, although the mode of inheritance is problematical because the affected females are sterile.

clude that there is a cause–and–effect relationship between the extra Y chromosome and violent behavior.

Testicular Feminization

ONE OF THE strangest sexual anomalies occurs in individuals who externally have typical female features, display feminine attitudes, and are reared as females, but are genetically males with a normal XY chromosome complement. The condition is known as testicular feminization. Affected individuals have well-developed breasts, but lack ovaries and never menstruate. Although they marry as females, they are infertile. The vagina comes to a blind end internally; a pair of undescended testes occupies the place of the missing ovaries. The Y chromosome apparently promotes the development of testes, but some factor prevents full realization of maleness.

The parents of such XY females are normal. Affected offspring occur in more than one generation, as shown in the pedigree in FIGURE 7–5. The pattern of inheritance points to transmission through the patient's mother of a single defective gene, either a recessive gene carried on the X chromosome or an autosomal dominant gene which is expressed only in XY individuals. The specific mode of inheritance is problematical inasmuch as the affected individual leaves no offspring.

The undescended testes produce large amounts of feminizing estrogens. The female secondary sexual characteristics will fail to develop if the testes are removed before puberty. The defective gene thus not only alters the male-determining role of the Y chromosome, but also somehow converts the testes into an organ directing the development of female secondary sexual characteristics.

Sex-Linked Inheritance

IT MUST NOT BE ASSUMED that the sex chromosomes are associated only with the sex of the individual. Genes for several traits which have no relation to sexual development are carried on the sex chromosomes, particularly the X. Those genes which are carried by the X chromosome are said to be sex-linked. Among the sex-linked genes are those responsible for hemophilia, red-green color blindness, and a form of muscular dystrophy.

The sex-linked genes are paired in the female since she has two X chromosomes. But the male has only one X chromosome and accordingly carries only a single, unpaired sex-linked gene. There is no corresponding gene on the Y chromosome. Thus, if the male carries a single defective X-borne gene, he is abnormal. If the given single gene is normal, he is normal.

The special features of sex-linked inheritance are seen in the transmission of hemophilia. This condition, often called "bleeder's disease," is a disorder of the blood in which a vital clotting factor is lacking, causing abnormally delayed clotting. Hemophilia is exhibited almost exclusively by males, who receive the defective gene from their mothers. The transmission of hemophilia is exemplified in the crosses illustrated in FIGURE 7-6. The normal X chromosome which contains the normal gene for proper clotting is indicated as a large X; the abnormal

INHERITANCE IN HEMOPHILIA

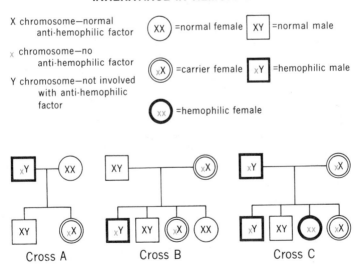

FIG. 7-6 INHERITANCE OF HEMOPHILIA. Males afflicted with hemophilia are sons of normal, but carrier, females. Hemophilic males do not transmit the defect to their children, but their daughters are carriers. Not all sons of carrier females are hemophilic; the expectation is that 50 percent of the sons will be normal and 50 percent hemophilic.

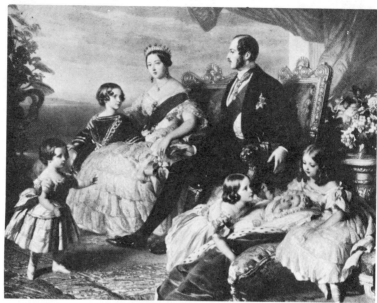

FIG. 7-7 QUEEN VICTORIA AND PRINCE ALBERT with their family in 1846, painted by Winterhalter. Queen Victoria's first two sons (at her *left*), Albert Edward (King Edward VII) and Alfred (Duke of Edinburgh), were not hemophilic. Of her first three daughters (at Prince Albert's *right*), the eldest, Victoria, is suspected of being a carrier of hemophilia. Her second daughter, Alice, was a carrier, and through her, hemophilia was transmitted into the Russian royal family. Her third daughter, Helena (the baby in the picture), was not a carrier.

gene-bearing X as a small x. If a hemophilic man (xY) marries a noncarrier woman (XX), all sons will be normal (XY) and all daughters will be carriers (xX). If a carrier woman (xX) marries a normal male (XY), there are four possibilities among the offspring (FIG. 7-6B). Each son has a 50-50 chance of being a victim, and each daughter has a 50-50 chance of being a carrier. The third mating illustrated (FIG. 7-6C) is an extremely remote one—that of a hemophilic male marrying a carrier female. Only from such a marriage can a hemophilic female arise (xx). A few hemophilic females have been recorded; some have married and given birth to hemophilic sons.

There is no known cure for hemophilia. The victim of hemophilia lives in constant danger of severe bleeding from the most minor wounds, such as a facial scratch or a tooth extraction. Hemorrhages can only be checked with transfusions of fresh whole blood (or plasma) or concentrates of the clotting protein known as antihemophilic globulin (AHG). The vast majority of hemophilics (about 80 percent) lack AHG: the other victims have been found to lack another clotting component, called plasma thromboplastin (PTC). This has led to the recognition of two forms of hemophilia, the classical type (Hemophilia A, deficiency of AHG or factor VIII) and the newly discovered type (Hemophilia B, deficiency of PTC or factor IX). Hemophilia B is also called the Christmas disease, after the surname of the first hemophilic B patient identified. The average life expectancy in both conditions is approximately 18 years. The National Hemophilic Foundation estimates that hemophilia affects about 100,000 Americans. About 80 percent of the known cases have a family history of "bleeders." The other 20 percent are "new" cases which have arisen from newly mutated genes in the X chromosome of the egg.

Hemophilia has been described in the ancient Hebrew Talmud, in the Bible, and in the dramatic stories of the royal families of Europe. Queen Victoria of England was the original carrier of the hemophilic gene (FIG. 7-7). The fateful gene apparently originated by mutation in Victoria herself. Her father, Edward Duke of Kent, was not a bleeder, and there is no evidence that her mother, the Duchess of Kent, was a carrier. One of Victoria's four sons was hemophilic and two (or possibly three) of her five daughters were carriers. Through her two carrier daughters, Alice and Beatrice, hemophilia was carried into the Russian and Spanish ruling families (FIG. 7-8). The last Czarevitch of Russia, Alexis, and the two sons of Alfonso XIII, the last king of Spain, suffered from hemophilia. The devastating influence of the fanatical monk Rasputin upon the Czarina and Czar Nicholas II came from his alleged hypnotic control of the disease in Alexis. The affliction of the Russian and Spanish crown princes played a significant role in the overthrow of the two dynasties.

The present British royal family has been spared the harmful hemophilic gene. Queen Elizabeth traces to Queen Victoria through three generations of male descendants (King Edward VII, King George V, and King George VI). None of them was hemophilic, nor is Prince Philip Mountbatten.

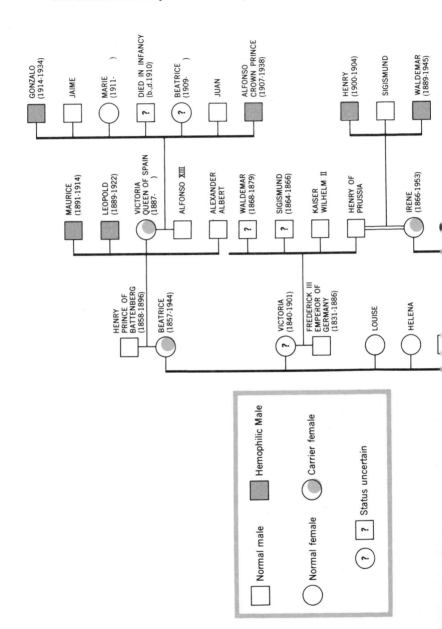

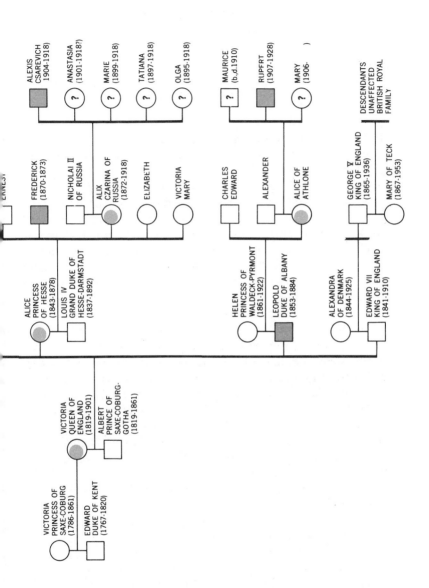

FIG. 7-8 PEDIGREE OF HEMOPHILIA in the royal families of Europe, traceable back to Queen Victoria of England.

Chapter 8

Sex Differences in Cells

IN THE PAST, there were no simple medical procedures to diagnose the existence of Turner's syndrome (XO) in the young girl before puberty. A short neck and broad chest in a stocky preadolescent girl aroused suspicion that she had a rudimentary ovary which would remain undeveloped throughout her life. Now the physician can scrape a few cells from the inside surface of the child's cheek, stain the cells, and detect the absence of one of the X chromosomes by simply examining the nuclei of the cells. This "sex chromatin test," as it is called, permits diagnosis of the XO female at an early age. She can be treated with female sex hormones to offset some of the sexual infantilism, although her sterile fate cannot be overcome.

The basis for the sex chromatin test emerged from a chance discovery in 1949 by Drs. Murray L. Barr and E. G. Bertram of the Medical School of the University of Western Ontario. In a routine examination of nerve cells of cats, they noted an unusually dark spot at the periphery of the nucleus of some of the cells (FIG. 8–1). The darkly stained body appeared only in the nuclei of cells from female cats. It was absent in the nerve cells of males. This small nuclear body that distinguished the sexes is called "sex chromatin," or after its discoverer, a Barr body. The Barr body was then shown to be present in female cells other than nerve cells, including the inner-cheek cells in humans.

Barr's discovery was followed by an announcement from London in 1954 that a sex difference could be detected in certain human white blood cells, the polymorphonuclear leucocytes. While studying the leucocytes of peripheral blood of a female patient, Drs. William M. Davidson and David R. Smith of King's College Hospital in London observed a roundish body attached by a thin stalk to one of the lobes of the nucleus (FIG. 8-1). This "drumstick," as they called it, is absent in the male and therefore provides an additional indicator of sex.

Both Barr bodies and drumsticks are seen in resting cells, in which the individual chromosomes are not distinguishable. Yet it appeared likely that these round bodies were related in some manner to the X chromosome of the female. That a relationship does exist became apparent from studies of individuals suffering from chromosomal sex anomalies.

Nuclear Sex and Chromosomal Anomalies

WHEN THE SEX CHROMATIN TEST was applied to patients with Klinefelter's syndrome (XXY), most of them were found to

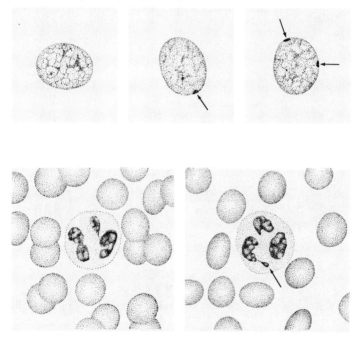

FIG. 8-1 THE BARR BODY, a small, darkly stained spot that distinguishes the sex: present once in the normal female *(top middle)*, twice in the triplo-X female *(top right)*, and absent in the male *(top left)*. THE DRUMSTICK, an additional indicator of sex: present as a roundish body in the normal female *(bottom right)* and absent in the normal male *(bottom left)*.

have a Barr body in the nucleus of the cheek cell as well as the drumstick lobule in the polymorphonuclear leucocyte. In other words, these patients, male in general appearance, have the "chromatin-positive" pattern of the normal female (XX). On the other hand, the majority of females with gonadal dysgenesis (Turner's syndrome, XO) were shown to be chromatin-negative. They lack Barr bodies and drumsticks, as does the normal male (XY).

It is thus evident that the presence of a Barr body or a drumstick is associated with the presence of two X chromo-

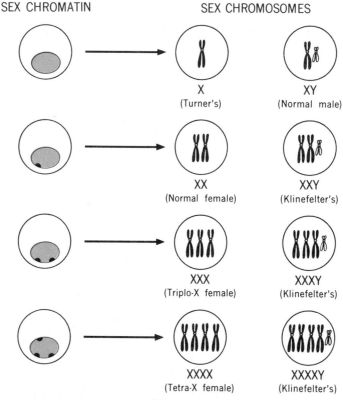

FIG. 8–2 RELATIONSHIP between the number of Barr bodies and the number of X chromosomes. The number of Barr bodies is always one less than the number of X chromosomes present in the individual.

somes, while the absence of sex chromatin is associated with the presence of a single X chromosome. From these considerations an important clinical generalization emerged: the finding of a sex-chromatin pattern that is contrary to the outward sex of the individual signifies sterility. As we have seen, a chromatin-negative pattern (normally male) in an anatomic female (Turner's syndrome) indicates the absence of a functional ovary. Similarly, a chromatin-positive pattern (normally female) in an anatomic male (Klinefelter's syndrome) signifies impairment of the testes.

Further studies in the 1950's revealed a striking relationship between the number of Barr bodies and the number of X chromosomes (FIG. 8–2). The cells of triplo-X females (XXX) contain two Barr bodies instead of one. Individuals with four X chromosomes—males (XXXXY) as well as females (XXXX)—have three Barr bodies. The maximum number of Barr bodies is therefore always one less than the number of X chromosomes present.

Sex Chromosomes in Somatic Cells

ALTHOUGH A RELATIONSHIP had been established between the number of Barr bodies and the number of sex chromosomes, it was still not clear as to what the Barr body itself represented. In the late 1950's the Japanese-born geneticist Dr. Susumu Ohno and his colleagues, at the City of Hope Medical Center in Duarte, California, made careful observations on dividing body cells of several kinds of animals, including the opossum, rat, and man. It will be recalled that the chromosomes first become visible as delicate threads during the prophase stage. In the prophase nuclei of female cells, Ohno and his colleagues noted that one thread was more compact than all other threads. Specifically, this thread, considered to be an X chromosome, was tightly coiled and deeply staining (FIG. 8–3). The other X chromosome was as lightly staining as the autosomes. The darkly stained, highly condensed X chromosome takes up a position against the nuclear membrane, and forms the Barr body. There is no doubt that the Barr body is derived from one of the X chromosomes, the deeply stained X.

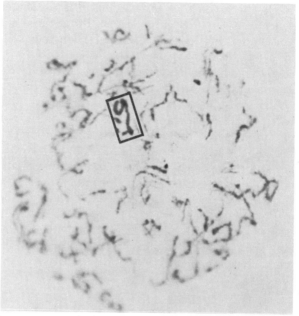

FIG. 8-3 PHOTOGRAPH OF FEMALE CHROMOSOMES showing one of the X chromosomes as contracted and dense. This darkly stained X chromosome is destined to form the Barr body. (Courtesy of Dr. Susumu Ohno, City of Hope Medical Center, California.)

Sex Chromatin in the Early Embryo

STUDIES IN 1957 by the embryologist Emil Witschi on preserved human embryos in the collections of the Carnegie Institution in Baltimore showed the chromatin-negative male and chromatin-positive female patterns in the heart cells of three-week-old embryos, before any visible development of the gonads. These observations were extended back in time to an earlier life of the embryo by Drs. T. W. Glenister and W. W. Park, both of whom independently were able to demonstrate the Barr body (the condensed X) in human female embryos immediately before, or shortly after, implantation in the uterus, when the embryo consists of several hundred cells.

Investigators then raised the question as to which one of the two X's of the embryo—the X contributed by the mother or the father's X—is relegated to the status of the dark Barr body. The evidence indicates that neither of the two is selected for the role. It is solely a matter of chance—the paternal X may become condensed in some cells, theoretically half the cells, and the maternal X in the remaining cells of the embryo. The outcome, as seen in FIGURE 8-4, is that the female is a genetic mosaic of paternal X's and maternal X's. The old tiresome cliché of the male about "crazy, mixed-up women" now merits attention.

The Lyon Hypothesis

IN THE EARLY 1960's, the British geneticist Mary F. Lyon formulated the intriguing theory that the condensed X of the female becomes genetically inactive early in embryonic development and remains a muted or silent partner of the functional X throughout life. The inactive X hypothesis, so brilliantly set forth, has become known as the Lyon hypothesis. The inactive X can be either the maternal X or the paternal X in different cells of the same female. Lyon marshaled evidence for her thesis from female mice that are heterozygous for sex-linked genes affecting coat color. The coat of certain heterozygotes consists of patches of normal dark color and mutant light color (FIG. 8-5). The Lyon hypothesis attributes this variegation to the early inactivation of the X chromosome carrying the normal gene in the cells of the mutant-colored

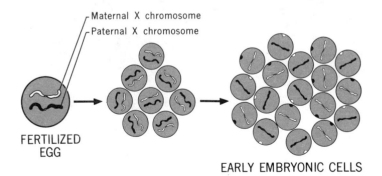

FIG. 8-4 DIAGRAMMATIC REPRESENTATION of the fate of one of the X chromosomes in an early female embryo. Either the maternal X or the paternal X may form the Barr body in a given female cell.

patches, and conversely, the suppression of the mutant X-borne gene in the cells of the normal-colored patches.

The Lyon hypothesis also provides an answer for an enigma that has long puzzled geneticists. Since the X chromosome carries genes that control the production of many chemical substances, particularly enzymes, then a female with a double dose of X chromosomes should produce twice as much of these enzymes as the male with one X. But she actually does not, nor could she if one of the X's is invariably inactivated.

In 1962, Dr. Ernest Beutler and his co-workers at the City of Hope Medical Center at Duarte, California, studied the red blood cells of females heterozygous for a recessive sex-linked gene that affects the production of a certain enzyme important

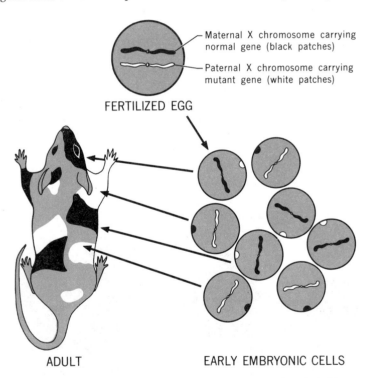

FERTILIZED EGG

Maternal X chromosome carrying normal gene (black patches)

Paternal X chromosome carrying mutant gene (white patches)

ADULT   EARLY EMBRYONIC CELLS

FIG. 8–5 THE LYON HYPOTHESIS. One of the X chromosomes is inactivated in some cells and the other X chromosome is inactivated in the other cells. The remaining functional X chromosome produces either a dark patch or a light patch. (Based on studies by Dr. Mary Lyon, Radiobiological Research Unit, England.)

in sugar metabolism, technically called glucose-6-phosphate dehydrogenase. The male either carries the normal gene on his sole X chromosome, in which case he produces the normal amount of the enzyme, or he carries the mutant gene and is accordingly unable to produce the enzyme at all. The male carrying the defective sex-linked gene is vulnerable to a potentially fatal anemia if he eats fava or broad beans or takes one of the modern antimalarial drugs, especially primaquine. The heterozygous female is not victimized since she bears both the normal and mutant gene. But Dr. Beutler found that the cells of the heterozygous female do not all uniformly produce the important enzyme. She contains rather a mixture of normal enzyme-producing cells and mutant enzyme-deficient cells, as if the normal X chromosome was inactivated in some cells and the mutant X chromosome in others.

Further substantiation of the inactive X hypothesis came from the laboratory of Dr. M. M. Grumbach, who found that the level of glucose-6-phosphate dehydrogenase activity is substantially the same in persons who have from one to four X chromosomes. This would follow from the Lyon hypothesis, since whatever the number of X chromosomes present in any individual, only a single one remains active. The Lyon hypothesis would also explain the curious finding that the XXXY variant of Klinefelter's syndrome is not more abnormal than

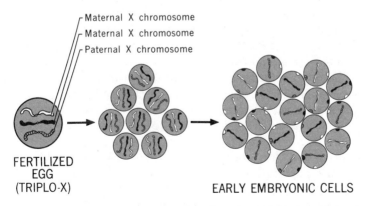

Maternal X chromosome
Maternal X chromosome
Paternal X chromosome

FERTILIZED
EGG
(TRIPLO-X)

EARLY EMBRYONIC CELLS

FIG. 8–6 DIAGRAMMATIC REPRESENTATION of the fate of two of the three X chromosomes in an early triplo-X embryo. The X chromosomes in excess of one shrivel into Barr bodies.

the XXY Klinefelter patient. In either case, only one X is functional. Similarly, triplo-X females are likely to be relatively free of defects since two of the three X chromosomes would assume the condensed state at about the time of implantation of the embryo (FIG. 8–6).

The Lyon hypothesis has not been proved beyond doubt. It is, however, reasonable and eminently plausible.

Sex Ratio

AS PREVIOUSLY STATED, the presence or absence of the Barr body can be demonstrated in human embryos at the time of implantation, a week or so after fertilization. The nuclear sex of the fetus can thus be established before it is born. Sex-chromatin studies have been carried out on fetal cells found in the amniotic fluid. A needle is inserted through the mother's abdomen to extract a sample of the amniotic fluid. The fetal cells, floating in the fluid, are then stained and examined for the presence or absence of the Barr body.

Many more males than females are undoubtedly conceived. The male-to-female sex ratio at fertilization has been variously estimated from 116:100 to as high as 160:100. However, spontaneous abortions occur more frequently among male than among female fetuses. The sex ratio at birth is 106 males to 100 females. The mortality rate among males is higher at all ages. The male to female ratio drops to 100:100 at age 20, and progressively declines thereafter to reach the staggering figure of 62:100 at age 85. There are no satisfactory explanations for the higher male mortality.

The reasons for the greater number of male conceptions are largely unkown. It appears unlikely that unequal numbers of X-bearing and Y-bearing sperms are produced, although this possibility cannot be discounted. More likely, the Y-bearing sperm is more viable than the X-bearing sperm, or more proficient in fertilization. It has been suggested that the Y-bearing sperm has a greater chance of reaching and penetrating the egg. The X chromosome is larger than the Y, and accordingly has a greater mass. Since velocity is dependent on mass, the sperm carrying the Y chromosome should be able to travel in the female reproductive canal at a greater speed with the same amount of energy than the sperm bearing the X chromosome. This explanation may be regarded as reasonable, although not proved.

Foreshadowing Sex

BIOLOGISTS TODAY are looking for the means to control sex prenatally. In a microscopic study of sperm specimens from hundreds of normal males, Dr. Landrum B. Shettles of Columbia University detected two distinct types of sperm cells. One kind, believed to be the X-bearing sperm, has an elongated, oval-shaped head, with the other, presumably the Y-bearing sperm, having a more compact, round head. Eventually, it may be possible to separate the two varieties in a test tube (before insemination), either on the basis of their differing electric charge or their difference in weight. The desired sperm cells can then be introduced by means of a syringe into the female during the period of ovulation. Parents in the near future may be afforded the opportunity to predetermine the sex of the unborn child.

Chapter 9

Maternal-Fetal Blood Incompatibility

FROM A BIOCHEMICAL STANDPOINT, one out of every eight marriages is a potentially dangerous mismatch. Babies born of such risky marriages may become victims of an infuriatingly small chemical difference in the blood cells of the parents. In these marriages, numbering 200,000 or more a year in the United States, the wife lacks a component in her red blood cells—a component called the Rh factor because it was first isolated in the rhesus monkey. She is said to be "Rh-negative." In contrast, the husband has the factor and is "Rh-positive."

The chemical difference in the couple seldom affects the first baby. But all future offspring are threatened if the first baby is Rh-positive; that is, if the infant's blood cells contain the Rh factor. When the Rh factor of the first baby enters the mother's blood stream, the Rh-negative mother reacts to the factor as if it were a foreign substance, or *antigen.* Her body's immune system produces a chemically active substance, or *antibody,* to attack the antigen, much in the same manner that antibodies fight off infectious bacteria. The mother, having produced antibodies, is said to be immunized (or sensitized) against her baby's blood cells.

The mother typically does not build up antibodies in sufficient strength to harm her first infant (FIG. 9–1). But the antibodies remain in her body, and may linger for many months or years. If the second baby is also Rh-positive, the mother may send enough antibodies into the developing child's blood stream to destroy or injure her unborn child. This condition of mother-child blood incompatibility is known variously as *erythroblastosis fetalis,* hemolytic disease of the newborn, or simply Rh disease. The disease results in 5,000 stillbirths every year in the United States alone, and burdens 20,000 newborn infants with anemia, heart failure, jaundice, or mental retardation.

Until recently, the only treatment was to replace the entire blood supply of the fetus with a transfusion of fresh blood, either immediately at birth (if the child was not stillborn) or before birth through the womb. This technique of exchange transfusion has been only partly successful. Now, after several years of testing, a "vaccine" has appeared on the scene which promises to protect *some* mothers from inflicting Rh disease on their babies.

Discovery of the Rh Factor

IN 1939, DR. PHILIP LEVINE and his colleague Dr. R. E. Stetson described the presence of an unusual type of antibody in the blood of a woman who had been given a transfusion of her husband's blood shortly after she had delivered a stillborn baby. She experienced chills and other symptoms of a severe antagonistic transfusion reaction even though she and her husband were presumably compatible as donor and recipient.

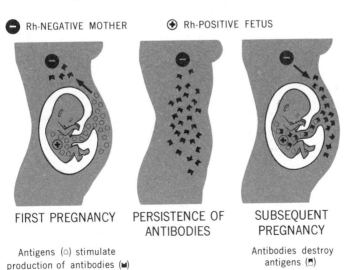

● Rh-NEGATIVE MOTHER   ⊕ Rh-POSITIVE FETUS

FIRST PREGNANCY   PERSISTENCE OF ANTIBODIES   SUBSEQUENT PREGNANCY

Antigens (○) stimulate production of antibodies (◣)

Antibodies destroy antigens (◙)

FIG. 9-1 Rh DISEASE in the newborn. The first baby is rarely harmed, but subsequent babies are potential victims of the mother's antibodies which are capable of destroying the infant's blood cells.

Levine and Stetson speculated that the woman had been stimulated to produce antibodies during her pregnancy by some unidentified antigen which the fetus had inherited from the father. When she later received blood from her husband, the antibodies already circulating in her blood stream agglutinated (clumped) her husband's cells. Evidently a new type of blood-group incompatibility had been found. No name was then assigned to the new antigen or its antibody.

About the same time, in another laboratory, Dr. Karl Landsteiner, Nobel laureate 1930 (1868–1943) and Dr. Alexander S. Wiener were studying the reactions of rabbits which had received injections of blood cells from rhesus monkeys. The rabbits responded by producing an antibody, previously undescribed, against a specific antigen in the blood cells of the monkeys. They called the antibody "anti-rhesus," or in shortened form, "anti-Rh." When anti-Rh was tested against human blood it was observed to react against the red cells of 85 percent of a large group of blood donors. These donors thus contained the Rh antigen and were designated Rh-positive. The other 15 percent who did not react to anti-Rh lacked the Rh antigen and were said to be Rh-negative. It was then quickly recognized that the anti-Rh induced in rabbits by Landsteiner and Wiener was the same as that recovered from the serum of mothers who had suffered severe transfusion reactions and, more particularly, of mothers who had given birth to infants with erythroblastosis.

By the close of 1941, the relationship of the Rh factor (or antigen) to erythroblastosis fetalis had become firmly established. Clinical records revealed that the mothers of erythroblastotic babies are always Rh-negative. The father and the child possess the Rh antigen that is absent in the mother. The cause of hemolytic disease of the newborn is the anti-Rh antibody produced by the mother in response to, and directed against, the Rh antigen of the blood cells of her own fetus.

Genetic and Clinical Aspects of Rh Disease

THE Rh ANTIGEN in the blood cell is controlled by a dominant gene, designated *R*. An Rh-positive person has the dominant gene, either in the homozygous *(RR)* or heterozygous *(Rr)* state. All Rh-negative individuals carry two recessive genes *(rr)* and are incapable of producing the Rh antigen.

The inheritance of the Rh antigen follows simple Mendelian laws (FIG. 9-2). A mother who is Rh-negative *(rr)* need not fear having Rh-diseased offspring if her husband is likewise Rh-negative *(rr)*. If the husband is heterozygous *(Rr)*, half of the offspring will be Rh-negative *(rr)* and none of these will be afflicted. The other half will be Rh-positive *(Rr)*, just like the father, and are potential victims of the disease. If the Rh-positive father is homozygous *(RR)*, then all the children will be Rh-positive *(Rr)* and potential victims. In essence, an Rh-positive child carried by an Rh-negative mother is the setting for possible, though not inevitable, trouble.

The chain of events leading to erythroblastosis fetalis begins with the inheritance by the fetus of the dominant *R* gene of the father. Rh antigens are produced in the red blood cells of the fetus. The fetal red cells bearing the Rh antigens escape

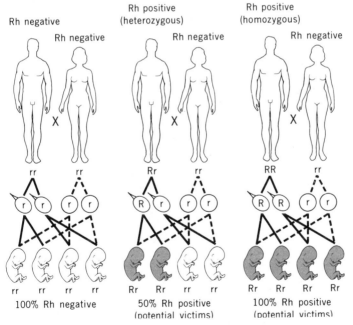

FIG. 9-2 SCHEME OF INHERITANCE of Rh Disease. An Rh-positive child carried by an Rh-negative mother is the setting for possible, though not inevitable, trouble.

through the placental barrier into the mother's circulation, and stimulate the production of antibodies (anti-R) against the Rh antigens on the fetal red cells. As stated earlier, the maternal antibodies almost never attain a sufficient concentration during the first pregnancy to harm the fetus. The firstborn infant is rarely affected, unless the mother has previously developed antibodies from having been transfused with Rh-positive blood or has had a prior pregnancy terminating in an abortion.

The mother's antibodies attach to the infant's red cells and cause destruction of the red cells. The fetus may die while in the womb or be born in critical condition from anemia. Se-

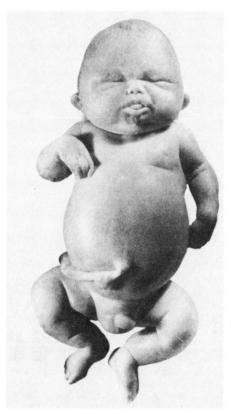

FIG. 9–3 GROSSLY MISSHAPEN infant suffering from Rh Disease. (From E. L. Potter, *Rh,* Year Book Medical Publishers, 1947.)

verely anemic infants are likely to develop heart failure. When the red cells hemolyze (break down), the hemoglobin liberated from the ruptured cells is transformed into a yellow pigment called bilirubin. The liver ordinarily would convert the bilirubin into harmless bile. But the amount of yellow bilirubin in the infant is unmanageable and accumulates in the blood, turning the plasma into an almost yellow-orange liquid. The infant is consequently deeply jaundiced—that is, the skin assumes a deep yellow-orange tint.

The grave danger to the infant lies in the prolonged exposure of the brain to high levels of bilirubin. Bilirubin has been shown to be highly toxic to the soft brain tissues; the brain may be permanently damaged. In the more seriously afflicted infants, the body tissues swell with abnormal amounts of fluid and the liver and spleen are enormously large (FIG. 9–3).

Another aspect of the condition, which has given it its name, is the presence of immature red cells (the erythroblasts) in the circulating blood. It is as if the liver and the spleen in an attempt to combat the severe anemic condition produce vast numbers of "unfinished" red blood cells. Unattended, erythroblastosis fetalis leads to stillborn or neonatal death. Many of the erythroblastotic babies are saved by exchange transfusion of Rh-negative blood; others, however, die despite treatment. Exchange transfusion is essentially a flushing-out process, whereby the infant's blood is gradually diluted with Rh-negative donated blood until at the end of the procedure most of the infant's circulating blood is problem-free.

The Rh gene has turned out to be more complex than initially envisioned. The Rh gene is not a single entity, nor is the Rh antigen a single uniform substance. There are several variant forms of the Rh gene, and a corresponding diversity of antigenic constitutions. This diversity need not concern us here. The most common antigen is the one that was first recognized, known more specifically now as Rh_o or D. It is the presence of Rh_o that is tested in ordinary clinical work.

Incidence of Rh Disease

AMONG CAUCASIANS in the United States, the incidence of Rh-negative persons is approximately 15 percent. In certain

European groups, such as the Basques in Spain, the frequency of Rh-negative individuals rises as high as 34 percent. Non-Caucasian populations are remarkably relatively free of Rh disease. The incidence of Rh-negative persons among the full-blooded American Indians, Eskimos, African Negro, Japanese, and Chinese is one percent or less. In contrast, the frequency of Rh negativity is high in the American Negro (nine percent), which reflects the historical consequences of intermarriages. The ancestry of the American Negro is approximately one-third Caucasian.

Approximately 13 percent of all marriages, or one out of every eight, are potentially dangerous with respect to erythroblastosis fetalis. However, only about one woman in 20 of the risky marriages does, in fact, produce an erythroblastotic infant. The reasons for this fortunately low observed incidence are not entirely clear. Apparently, differences in the ease of sensitization exist among Rh-negative women. The Rh antigen of the fetus may fail to get through the placenta, or some Rh-negative mothers are incapable of responding to the antigen. The low occurrence may also reflect a peculiar protective role of the "ABO" blood groups in reducing the risk of Rh incompatibility. This curious interaction requires an understanding of the ABO blood system.

ABO Incompatibility

THE Rh FACTOR is not the only antigen that a red blood cell may possess on its surface. Red blood cells may carry as well two other major antigens, called A and B. The A and B factors were discovered in the early 1900's by the Austrian scientist Karl Landsteiner. His discovery led to the identification of the four familiar major human blood groups or types—A, B, AB, and O.

A person might possess one or the other antigen, in which case he would be either type A or type B, or contain both antigens (type AB), or have neither antigen (type O). There are two corresponding antibodies in the serum of the blood, anti-A and anti-B. These antibodies occur naturally in the body and do not arise as the result of immunization.

A person does not have the antibody that will destroy his

own cells (TABLE 9-1). Stated another way, a person does not have the antibody corresponding to his own antigen. He may, however, possess the antibody which reacts against the antigen possessed by another person. For example, type A individuals lack anti-A but contain the antibody against B. This knowledge provides the basis for the successful transfusion of blood between individuals. The cardinal rule is to avoid introducing antigens that can be destroyed (or agglutinated) by antibodies in the serum of the recipient. Type O individuals are the acknowledged "universal donors" since they contain no antigens that could be acted upon by the recipient's antibodies. Type AB persons lack both antibodies and accordingly can receive blood from persons of all types without fear of destroying the cells contributed by the donor.

TABLE 9-1.

ABO Blood Groups				
Group	Genotype	Antigens in Cells	Antibodies in Serum	Can Donate Blood to:	Can Receive Blood from:
A	$I^A I^A$ or $I^A i$	A	anti-B	A, AB	A, O
B	$I^B I^B$ or $I^B i$	B	anti-A	B, AB	B, O
AB	$I^A I^B$	A & B	none	AB	A, B, AB, O
O	ii	none	anti-A & anti-B	A, B, AB, O	O

The ABO blood groups are governed by three contrasting genes, designated I^A, I^B and i. Although three genes are involved, a person can possess only two of the genes (TABLE 9-1). If a person inherits the I^A and I^B genes, one from each parent, he will have type AB blood. A double dose of the i gene results in an O type. A person belonging to blood group A either has the I^A gene in homozygous condition $(I^A I^A)$ or in association with the i gene $(I^A i)$. The I^B gene in the homozygous state $(I^B I^B)$ or heterozygous condition $(I^B i)$ results in the B blood type.

It may happen that the fetus contains an A or B antigen (inherited from the father) that is not present in the mother herself. The mother, for example, may be type O and her baby may be type A. The mother in this case would carry the naturally occurring antibodies in her serum, anti-A and anti-B. The mother's anti-A antibody would destroy the infant's red cells carrying the A antigen. Erythroblastosis due to anti-A (or anti-B) may occur in the firstborn. However, the disease is much milder than that caused by anti-Rh, and occurs less often (about one in 1,000 pregnancies). Apparently, anti-A and anti-B cross the placenta less readily than anti-Rh. Nevertheless, ABO disease is at least twice as common as Rh disease. The principal clinical manifestation of ABO disease is jaundice, indicative of an elevated bilirubin content in the infant's serum. These infants are as equally incompetent to handle the excess bilirubin as are the Rh-diseased infants, and the treatment is the same—namely, exchange transfusion.

TABLE 9–2.

ABO Groups of Mothers and Their Babies

Mother's Type	Antibodies in Mother's Serum	Types of Incompatible Babies	Types of Compatible Babies
A	anti-B	B, AB	O, A
B	anti-A	A, AB	O, B
AB	none	none	A, B, AB
O	anti-A & anti-B	A, B	O

Theoretically, 20 percent of all babies have ABO blood types that are potentially incompatible with the mother's. An examination of TABLE 9–2 reveals that type AB women do not have "incompatible" babies and that type O babies are always "compatible." Examples of "incompatible" marriages are shown in FIGURE 9–4.

A disquieting finding in recent years is that anti-A and anti-B appear to attack the fetus early in pregnancy, resulting in abortion or miscarriage. It has been observed that spontaneous abortion before the sixth month of pregnancy occurs more often among type O women married to men of type A or B than among A or B women married to O men. In terms of pregnancies terminating prematurely, ABO incompatibility looms more frightening than Rh incompatibility.

Ironically, ABO incompatibility between mother and fetus may have beneficial consequences. We remarked earlier that the actual observed incidence of Rh disease is much lower than that theoretically expected. In 1943, Dr. Philip Levine called attention to the fact that infants of Rh-negative, type O

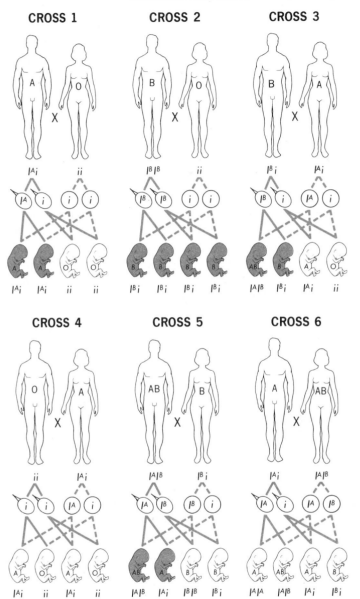

FIG. 9–4 BABIES of certain marriages have blood types that are potentially incompatible with that of the mother. Blood type O babies are never in danger, and type AB mothers can never harm their infants. Babies in potential danger are highlighted.

mothers develop Rh disease less often than those of A or B, Rh-negative mothers. The evidence indicates that the maternal anti-A and anti-B antibodies destroy the child's Rh-positive red cells when they invade the Rh-negative mother's blood stream. Thus, the incompatible fetal cells are rapidly eliminated before they have the opportunity to sensitize the mother. Strange as it may seem, then, the ABO incompatibility protects the mother and child against a simultaneous Rh incompatibility.

The Control of Rh Disease

ALTHOUGH FETAL CELLS cross the placenta throughout pregnancy, they enter the maternal circulation in much larger numbers during delivery, when the placental vessels rupture. It is now generally conceded that sensitization of the mother takes place shortly after the delivery of the first Rh-positive child. In the 1960's Drs. Vincent Freda and John Gorman at the Columbia-Presbyterian Medical Center in New York and Dr. William Pollack at the Ortho Research Foundation in New Jersey sought the means to suppress the production of antibodies in mothers who had recently delivered an Rh-positive infant. Experiments performed 50 years earlier by the distinguished American bacteriologist, Dr. Theobald Smith (1859–1934), furnished an important clue to the solution. In 1909, Smith arrived at the general principle that "passive" immunity can prevent "active" immunity. That is, an antibody given passively by injection can inhibit the recipient from producing its own active antibody.

After five years of experimentation and testing, Drs. Freda, Gorman, and Pollack successfully developed a "vaccine" consisting of a blood fraction (gamma globulin) rich in Rh antibodies. Injected into the blood stream of the Rh-negative mother no later than three days after the birth of her first Rh-positive child, the globulin-Rh antibody preparation suppresses the mother's antibody-making activity. Several hundred mothers have already received the preparation; none has formed active antibodies. More impressively some of them have now delivered a second Rh-positive baby and none of the babies were afflicted with Rh disease. The evidence is overwhelming that the vaccine is effective.

Unfortunately, the vaccine offers no hope for mothers who have already acquired their own permanent antibodies by earlier pregnancies or by previous transfusion of Rh-positive blood. Moreover, the inoculation of the globulin-Rh antibody must be repeated after each subsequent Rh-positive pregnancy. But this is a small inconvenience for the gift of a normal baby.

Chapter 10

Gene-Enzyme Defects

EARLY IN THIS CENTURY, the English physician Archibald E. Garrod (1857–1936) reported several cases of a peculiar disorder in which his patients excreted "black urine." The first alarming sign of the anomaly occurs during infancy when the mother notices that her baby's diapers are darkly stained. The black color is due to a chemical substance, first called "alkapton" and now positively identified as homogentisic acid. Urine containing homogentisic acid, in contact with air, gradually turns dark.

Normally homogentisic acid is converted into another substance in the body and does not appear in the urine. But infants afflicted with alkaptonuria (derived from "alkapton") are incapable of transforming homogentisic acid into other products, and abnormal amounts of this substance are eliminated in the urine. The condition is harmless in early life, but as the child grows older, black pigment slowly accumulates in various tissues of the body. The deposition of pigment in the joints of the knee, shoulder, and hips may be followed by degenerative changes leading to incapacitating arthritis and death. Although rare and sporadic, about 200 cases of alkaptonuria have been reported in the world literature. Most of the reported cases have been in Caucasians.

In 1902, Garrod observed that alkaptonuria occurred more often in families in which there were consanguineous marriages. Moreover, the parents of afflicted infants were generally unaffected. From these considerations, Garrod postulated that alkaptonuria was caused by a defective recessive gene, which manifests its detrimental effect when the child inherits one abnormal gene from each of his parents. He emphasized that alkaptonuria was an inherited biochemical disease, or, as he called it, an "inborn error of metabolism."

In 1908, Garrod expanded his ideas. He theorized that the defective gene prevents the formation of a particular enzyme. In other words, a single vital enzyme is missing in alkaptonuric patients. An enzyme is a complex protein which permits or hastens the conversion of one substance (or substrate) to a new substance (or product). As seen in FIGURE 10-1, the normal gene leads to the formation of an enzyme that transforms homogentisic acid to another product, acetoacetic acid. In an alkaptonuric patient, the enzyme is absent or deficient and homogentisic acid accumulates since its conversion to acetoacetic acid is blocked or hindered. The accumulation of homogentisic acid leads to a pathological condition.

Important as Garrod's ideas have proved to modern medicine, they were not recognized as such by his colleagues of the day. His theory that an "inborn error of metabolism" resulted

NORMAL PERSON

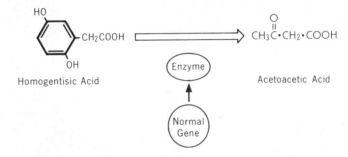

ALCAPTONURIC PERSON

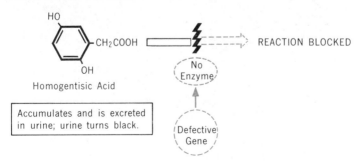

FIG. 10-1 ALKAPTONURIA, an inherited biochemical disease resulting from the absence of a vital enzyme.

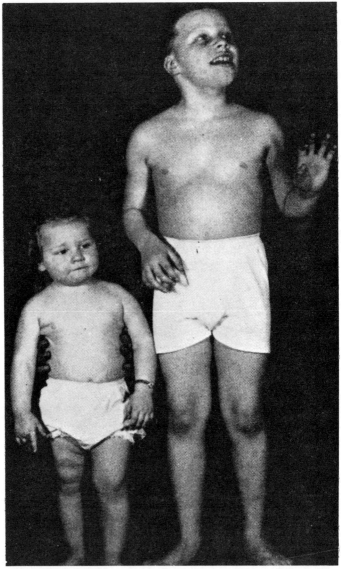

FIG. 10-2 SIBLINGS, ages 2 and 8 years, both suffering from phenylketonuria. The younger child is fair-skinned and has blond hair, characteristic of the majority of phenylketonuric patients. A small number of patients, like the older child, have dark hair. (Courtesy of Dr. Norman Kretchmer, Stanford University School of Medicine, California.)

from the absence of an enzyme fell on deaf ears. Verification came, however, in the 1940's from experiments performed on the pink bread mold by 1958 Nobel prize winners G. W. Beadle and Edward L. Tatum, then at the California Institute of Technology. They found that mutation of a particular gene blocks a particular metabolic reaction leading to the eventual production of a vital amino acid, with the consequence that the mold is unable to survive unless "fed" the essential amino acid. Beadle and Tatum set forth with special clarity and thoroughness the "one gene—one enzyme" concept, which states that each gene controls the formation of a single enzyme and thereby of a single metabolic reaction. In recent years, this concept has proved invaluable to the understanding of inherited human anomalies.

Phenylketonuria

ONE OF THE best known of the inherited biochemical diseases is phenylketonuria, abbreviated PKU. The first case of PKU was described by the Norwegian physician-chemist Asbjörn Fölling in 1934. Persons suffering from PKU are mentally retarded, usually so severely that they are institutionalized. They frequently have a light complexion (blondish hair and bluish eyes) because the production of brown-black pigment (melanin) is impaired (FIG. 10-2). Most affected individuals also have postural peculiarities, convulsive or jerky movements, and an indisputable body odor, described as "musty" or "barny." Phenylketonuric individuals have a short life expectancy; less than 1 out of 4 live beyond 30 years of age. The incidence of PKU has been estimated at one in 25,000 births. The disability occurs most often among northern Europeans and least frequently among Jews, Negroes, and Orientals.

Shortly after birth, the affected infant has an unusually high concentration of phenylalanine in the blood. Phenylalanine, an essential amino acid, is required for the manufacture of most proteins of the body. Phenylalanine is normally converted to a slightly different amino acid, tyrosine, which is involved in several metabolic pathways, including the formation of pigment. In 1953, the New York physician Dr. George Jervis found that PKU infants are deficient in a liver enzyme (phenylalanine hydroxylase) that converts phenylalanine into tyrosine. Phenylalanine thus accumulates in the body fluids and tissues in large quantities. The increased concentration of phenylalanine leads, in turn, to an increased rate of formation of phenylpyruvic acid, which is excreted in the urine (FIG. 10–3). Excess phenylpyruvic acid in sweat accounts for the strange body odor of PKU patients.

It is not the lack of tyrosine that produces the abnormal consequences, but rather the excessive amounts of phenylalanine. High levels of phenylalanine are damaging to the rapidly

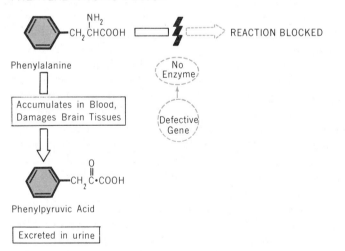

FIG. 10–3 PHENYLKETONURIA (PKU), an inherited biochemical disease resulting from the absence of a vital enzyme.

developing brain tissues of the infant in early life. After six months, the afflicted infant shows definite signs of mental retardation.

In 1961, Dr. Robert Guthrie of the Buffalo Medical School Children's Hospital devised a sensitive and reliable blood test to detect abnormal levels of phenylalanine in the infant during the first few days of life. Only a few drops of blood from the infant's heel are required to detect PKU. The Guthrie blood test or some modification of it has become mandatory in many hospitals in the United States. There are now indications that, although rare, the incidence of PKU may be greater than had been previously estimated. Approximately one in 10,000 newborn infants tested nationally in the early 1960's was found to be phenylketonuric.

Many of the newborn infants afflicted with PKU, if treated, have a chance to develop normally. Treatment of PKU has been directed toward reducing the intake of phenylalanine in the diet. In 1954, Drs. H. Bickel, J. Gerrard, and E. M. Hickmans devised a synthetic diet rich in the necessary proteins but low in content of phenylalanine. Although additional investigations are needed, the results have thus far been encouraging. Many phenylketonuric children who received the special diet early in life (from two months of age onward) have shown marked improvement in both physical and mental development. When the diet is discontinued, patients typically suffer a relapse.

The administration of a low phenylalanine diet early in the infant's life is especially important. The earlier the special diet is introduced, the more beneficial the effect. The crucial enzyme (phenylalanine hydroxylase) develops after birth, or at least is not normally active before birth. Thus, the phenylketonuric infant at birth has not sustained any damage to the brain. The key to successful treatment is to curtail the potentially harmful substrate (phenylalanine) before it has an opportunity to accumulate in the infant.

In the vast majority of families with phenylketonuric offspring, the parents are normal and are often related. The normal parents are heterozygous carriers of a defective recessive gene that inhibits the production of the enzyme phenylalanine hydroxylase. A child who inherits a double dose of the

TABLE 10-1

Risk of Phenylketonuric (PKU) Offspring in Various Marriages*

Marital partners A — Carrier status	A — Chances of carrying gene	Marital partners B — Carrier status	B — Chances of carrying gene	Theoretical frequency of affected children if both partners were carriers	Chances of affected children from such a mating
Unknown	1 in 80	Unknown	1 in 80	1 in 4	1 in 25,600
Unknown	1 in 80	Normal sibling of phenylketonuric	2 in 3	1 in 4	1 in 480
Unknown	1 in 80	Parent of phenylketonuric	1	1 in 4	1 in 320
Unknown	1 in 80	Phenylketonuric	1	1 in 2	1 in 160
Normal sibling of phenylketonuric	2 in 3	Normal sibling of phenylketonuric	2 in 3	1 in 4	1 in 9
Normal sibling of phenylketonuric	2 in 3	Parent of phenylketonuric	1	1 in 4	1 in 6
Normal sibling of phenylketonuric	2 in 3	Phenylketonuric	1	1 in 2	1 in 3
Parent of phenylketonuric	1	Parent of phenylketonuric	1	1 in 4	1 in 4
Parent of phenylketonuric	1	Phenylketonuric	1	1 in 2	1 in 2
Phenylketonuric	1	Phenylketonuric	1	1	1

*Calculated on prevalence rate of disease as approximately 1 in 25,000.

faulty recessive gene is not able to manufacture the enzyme.

The number of carriers of the faulty gene is about one in 80. Thus, the probability that two carriers from the general population will marry is one in 6,400 (80 × 80). If both marriage partners were carriers, then theoretically one of every four children would be afflicted with PKU. The first probability figure (one in 6,400) multiplied by the second probability figure (one in four) gives the total chance for affected children from this union, or one in 25,600. However, this probability is increased enormously if two normal individuals marry, both of whom had heterozygous carrier parents. The marital partners would each have a two-thirds chance of being carriers themselves, and the risk of affected children from such a marriage would be one in nine! Calculations of the risk of PKU in offspring from different types of marriages are shown in TABLE 10–1.

Recent studies indicate that the heterozygous carriers are distinguishable by chemical test from normal homozygous persons. Heterozygous individuals possess less than the normal amount of phenylalanine oxidase. Accordingly, an individual can now be tested to determine whether he harbors the defective recessive gene that can be passed on to his offspring.

The Phenylalanine Deficiencies

PHENYLALANINE IS THE starting point for a chain of chemical reactions essential in the metabolism of man. Connected with this chain of chemical reactions are four inherited defects, three of which we have already mentioned: alkaptonuria, phenylketonuria, albinism (see chapter 4), and tyrosinosis. Only one case of tyrosinosis has come to the attention of medical scientists. The disorder was recognized in a 49-year-old Russian who excreted abnormal amounts of p-hydroxyphenylpyruvic acid in the urine (FIG. 10–4).

Each of the four metabolic disorders results from a block at a different point in the same chain of chemical reactions beginning with phenylalanine. The locations of the enzymatic blocks in the overall scheme of metabolism of phenylalanine are shown in FIGURE 10–4. It still impresses medical scientists

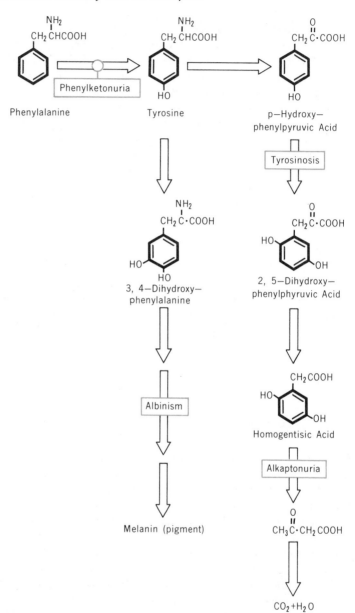

FIG. 10-4 FOUR INHERITED METABOLIC DISORDERS, each resulting from an enzymatic block at a different point in the chain of chemical reactions beginning with phenylalanine.

that four unusual disorders are linked to the metabolism of one amino acid.

Galactosemia

ONE OF THE most extraordinary inborn errors of metabolism is galactosemia, a condition in which the breast-fed infant is "poisoned" by the mother's milk. Afflicted infants are unable to utilize the kind of sugar, called galactose, that is found in milk. Galactose ordinarily is converted to glucose and, eventually, to energy. In affected infants, galactose is not transformed and accumulates in the blood. The infant suffers from malnutrition, becomes severely retarded mentally, and develops cataracts. Characteristically the liver becomes grossly enlarged. Unattended, the infant usually dies. More than forty cases of this disorder have been reported.

In 1956, Vernon Schwartz and his co-workers made the important observation that galactosemia resulted from a block in the conversion of the phosphate compound of galactose (galactose 1-phosphate) to glucose 1-phosphate. This was followed by the demonstration a year later by Herman Kalckar and his collaborators at the National Institutes of Health in Bethesda, Maryland, that the enzyme for this particular reaction was deficient. In turn, the absence of the enzyme is the consequence of a single defective recessive gene. In all cases of affected infants, both parents have proved to be heterozygous carriers. The heterozygous state can now be detected by simple chemical tests.

If the diagnosis of galactosemia is made before the disease is too far advanced, nearly all the symptoms of the disease disappear if galactose is excluded from the diet of the infant. The liver returns to normal size, nausea and vomiting cease, and nutrition and growth improve markedly. Unfortunately, unless therapy of a galactose-free diet is instituted promptly at birth, there is usually no recovery from the mentally retarded state.

Errors of Metabolism

GALACTOSEMIA VIVIDLY ILLUSTRATES the interplay of genetic factors and environmental factors. The defective recessive gene, when homozygous, is expressed only under certain environmental conditions. The particular environment happens to be the usual or normal one, since galactose is a main component of milk. Thus, under ordinary circumstances, all homozygous recessive offspring are vulnerable to galactosemia. However, if the environment is modified—that is, if galactose is eliminated from the diet—the disorder is curtailed or prevented. The individual will, of course, continue to lack the ability to manufacture the appropriate enzyme and remain always intolerant of galactose.

The modification of the diet is not the panacea for inborn errors of metabolism. It should be possible, theoretically, to cure metabolic errors either by transplanting cells capable of synthesizing the missing enzyme or by replacing the defective gene itself. The latter possibility is not preposterous or abstruse. Indeed, in December 1969, a team of Harvard researchers, led by Dr. Jonathan Beckwith, achieved the historic goal of isolating for the first time pure genes of living matter. The genes were removed from viruses, but this remarkable feat of isolating the gene itself paves the way to the repair or replacement of defective human genes and the elimination of their tragic consequences.

Chapter 11

Molecular Diseases

IN 1910, THE AMERICAN PHYSICIAN James B. Herrick (1861–1954) presented his findings of a peculiar blood disorder at the annual meeting of the Association of American Physicians. His report elicited little interest or comment. It consisted of a six-year study of an anemic West Indian Negro student residing in Chicago. The patient's blood was described as containing "peculiar elongated and sickle-shaped red corpuscles." The twisted appearance of the red blood cells is illustrated in FIGURE 11–1. The Negro patient was kept under ob-

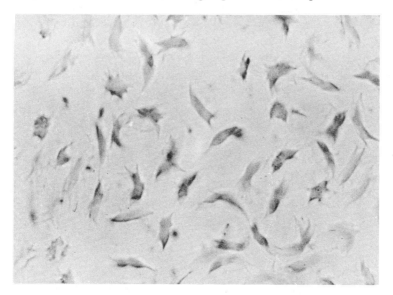

FIG. 11–1 PECULIARLY FLATTENED shape of red blood cells of an individual suffering from sickle-cell anemia. Red blood cells are normally spherical in appearance. (Courtesy of Dr. Norman Woody, Tulane University School of Medicine.)

servation for six years, during which time he displayed many of the distressing symptoms we now recognize as typical of the disease, called sickle-cell anemia. The bizarre-shaped red cells are fragile and clog small blood vessels. The obstruction of circulation leads in turn to the necrosis (death) of various tissues. The victim may suffer from pneumonia as a result of lung damage, rheumatism from muscle and joint deterioration, heart disease, and kidney failure. Inflammation of the soft tissues of the hands (and feet) is a frequent complication (FIG. 11–2). Physicians can provide care for the patient, but there is no cure. Affected persons rarely reach adult life.

This terrifying anomaly, which occurs predominantly in Negroes, was shown in the late 1940's by the human geneticist J. V. Neel of the University of Michigan to be inherited as a simple Mendelian recessive character. Then, in 1949, the distinguished chemist and Nobel laureate Linus Pauling and his co-workers made the important discovery that the defective recessive gene alters the configuration of the hemoglobin molecule, the oxygen-carrying component of the red corpuscle. This finding ushered in an entire new field of investigation in hu-

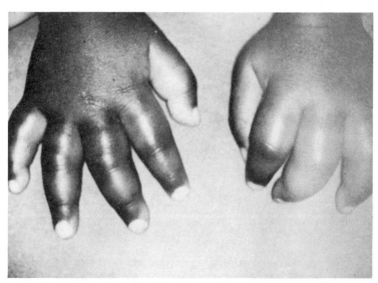

FIG. 11–2 INFLAMED FINGERS of a Negro youngster suffering from sickle-cell anemia. (Courtesy of Dr. Norman Woody, Tulane University School of Medicine.)

man biochemical genetics, culminating in a basic understanding of the role played by genes in the synthesis of vital body proteins.

Inheritance of Sickle-Cell Anemia

SICKLE-CELL ANEMIA results when the abnormal recessive gene is inherited in double dose *(aa)*. Heterozygous carriers of the sickle-cell gene *(Aa)* typically show no ill effects. However, under special conditions such as that encountered at high altitude, the blood cells develop a mildly sickled appearance. The benign heterozygous state is referred to as sickle-cell trait. The sickling phenomenon does not occur at all in individuals homozygous for *AA*.

Sickle-cell anemia is one of the most serious illnesses of Negro children. In fact, sickle-cell anemia is about six times more common than the next most common long-term illness of Negro children (diabetes). Very few individuals homozygous for the sickling gene survive to reproductive age. The sickling gene is particularly prevalent in the tropical zone of Africa. In some African communities the incidence of the sickle-cell trait may be as high as 40 percent. Such high frequencies can be understood only if there exists a special compensatory mechanism which replenishes the continual loss of the sickling gene resulting from the early death of homozygotes. Field work undertaken in Africa in 1949 by the British geneticist Anthony Allison revealed that the incidence of the sickle-cell trait is high in regions where malignant malaria is widespread. Carriers of the sickle-cell trait actually enjoy an immunity against malignant (tertian) malaria which is not shared by the normal homozygote. The sickle-cell trait protects infants against malarial infection. The protective effect of sickle-cell trait explains the persistence of an otherwise disadvantageous sickling gene.

The frequency of the sickling gene should be relatively low in malaria-free areas, where the positive advantage of the heterozygous sickle-cell trait is lost. The frequency of the sickling gene has fallen to low levels in the Negro population of the United States. The frequency of the sickle-cell trait among American Negroes is only about 8 percent. The incidence at birth of the disabling sickle-cell anemia in the United States is estimated at two per 1,000 infants.

Sickle-Cell Hemoglobin

IN 1949, DR. LINUS PAULING presented evidence that the hemoglobin molecule in sickle-cell anemia patients is abnormal. Pauling and his associates used the then relatively new technique of electrophoresis, which characterizes proteins according to the manner in which they move in an electric field. The hemoglobin molecule travels toward the positive pole. The speed of migration of the sickle cell's hemoglobin differs from that of normal hemoglobin; it moves slower than the normal molecule. The red corpuscles of heterozygous carriers were found to contain both kinds of hemoglobin—the normal type (designated hemoglobin A, or Hb A) and the sickle-cell anemia variety (Hb S)—in nearly equal quantities. The sickle-cell gene thus leads to some peculiarity in the synthesis of hemoglobin. In the heterozygote, the normal gene apparently functions independently of the defective gene, and two lines of synthesis—abnormal and normal—proceed. Apparently, then, there is a direct relation between the genes present and the kinds of hemoglobin formed.

It remained for Vernon Ingram at Cambridge University to ascertain how the hemoglobin molecule is altered by the aber-

Normal hemoglobin

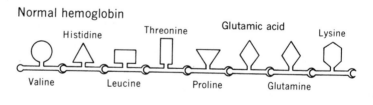

Sickle cell hemoglobin

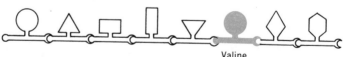

FIG. 11–3 THE SIMPLE SUBSTITUTION of a single amino acid, glutamine by valine, in a small section of the hemoglobin molecule is responsible for the abnormal sickling of the human red blood cell. (Based on studies by Dr. Vernon Ingram.)

rant gene. In 1956, Ingram ingeniously succeeded in breaking down hemoglobin, a large protein molecule, into several components (peptide fragments), each containing short sequences of identifiable amino acids (the basic units of protein). Normal hemoglobin and sickle-cell hemoglobin yielded the same array of peptide fragments, with a single exception. In one of the peptide fragments of sickle-cell hemoglobin, the amino acid glutamic acid had been replaced at one point in the chain by valine (FIG. 11-3). The sole difference in chemical composition between normal and sickle-cell hemoglobin is the substitution of a single amino acid among several hundred. The fatal effect of sickle-cell anemia is thus traceable to an exceedingly slight alteration in the structure of a protein molecule. How this minor alteration in the protein molecule arises brings us to the study of the chemical nature of the gene.

Chemical Nature of the Gene

PROTEINS, SUCH AS HEMOGLOBIN, are found in the cytoplasm of the cell. Yet the genes which control protein synthesis are in the nucleus. It had earlier been confidently assumed that proteins are manufactured in the nucleus and transported to the cytoplasm. However, the dramatic achievements in the last decade have made it convincingly clear that a genetic messenger migrates from the nucleus to the cytoplasm and there directs protein synthesis.

The genetic messenger is derived from two coiled chemical chains, known as deoxyribonucleic acid, or DNA. The DNA molecule is essentially a strand of genes. The unveiling of the chemical architecture of the DNA molecule and its recognition as the chemically active portion of the genes constitute one of the finest triumphs of modern science.

The Double Helix

THE TWO SCIENTISTS who had worked together in the early 1950's to solve the riddle of DNA were Francis H. C. Crick, the young biophysicist at Cambridge University, and James D. Watson, an American student of virology who was then in attendance at Cambridge on a post-doctoral fellowship to study chemistry. With the invaluable aid of X-ray pictures of DNA crystals prepared by Maurice H. F. Wilkins, the biophysicist at King's College in London, Watson and Crick built an elegant model in metal of DNA's configuration. The inspired model, now universally accepted, won Watson, Crick, and Wilkins the coveted Nobel Prize for Medicine and Physiology in 1962.

A remarkable feature of DNA is its simplicity. The DNA molecule is shaped like a twisted ladder (FIG. 11–4). The two parallel strands of the ladder are twisted about each other somewhat like the supporting frameworks of a spiral staircase. The twisted supports of the ladder are made up of phosphate and sugar compounds, endlessly repeated. Each rung of the

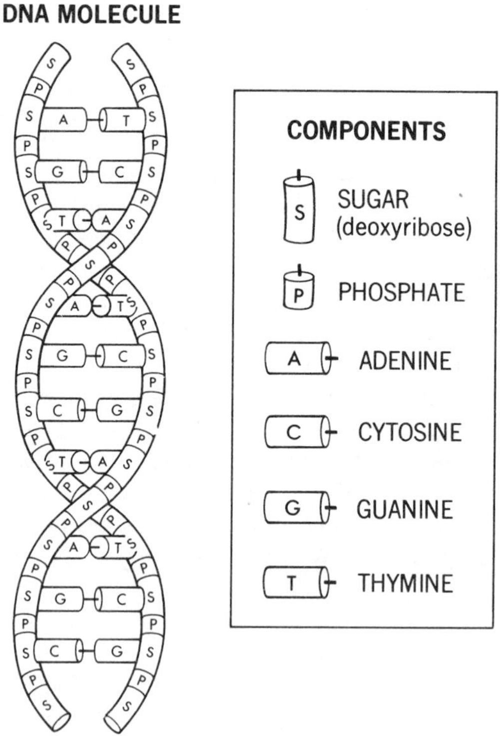

DNA MOLECULE

COMPONENTS

S — SUGAR (deoxyribose)

P — PHOSPHATE

A — ADENINE

C — CYTOSINE

G — GUANINE

T — THYMINE

FIG. 11–4 THE MASTER CHEMICAL OF LIFE, the double-stranded, ladderlike deoxyribonucleic acid (DNA).

ladder is made up of one pair of specific nitrogen-containing ring compounds, or nitrogenous bases. There are two classes of nitrogenous bases, the purines and the pyrimidines. Each rung or step consists of one purine coupled by hydrogen bonds to one pyrimidine. The purine called adenine (A) is normally joined with the pyrimidine called thymine (T) to constitute what may be termed a "base-pair" rung. Another purine, guanine (G) is typically linked with the pyrimidine cytosine (C) to form another base-pair rung. These two types of paired bases (A-T and G-C) are arranged in certain sequences in different chromosomes, and each gene owes its unique character to a specific order or arrangement of the base-pair rungs. It is the bases that determine the genetic message that DNA carries. A gene is a linear sequence of at least a thousand bases.

When a cell divides, its nucleus divides and, within the nucleus, each chromosome is replicated. Each gene accordingly has to make a copy of itself. In 1957, Nobel Prize winner Arthur Kornberg showed in principle that the DNA molecule simply unzips. The two parallel strands of the ladder split down the middle, breaking the hydrogen bonds that held together the paired bases. Each half rung on each half ladder then proceeds to attract new base units from its surrounding environment, so that eventually each half ladder will look like the old whole ladder. The original double helix thus produces two exact replicas of itself.

The Language of Life

PROTEINS ARE COMPOSED OF 20 basic building blocks, the amino acids, arranged in a long chain, called a polypeptide. The polypeptide chain may be several hundred amino acids in length. The properties of any protein are determined by the number, identity, and sequences of its amino acid blocks.

If DNA controls the synthesis of protein, then the four bases (A, C, G, and T) must be sufficient to determine the arrangements of the 20 different kinds of amino acids. In 1954, the theoretical physicist George Gamow (1904–1968) suggested that the four bases constitute a sort of four-letter alphabet or code. Each amino acid is dictated by one sequence of three bases in the original DNA molecule. As an example, the sequence adenine-adenine-guanine (AAG) in the DNA molecule might designate that the amino acid glutamic acid is to be incorporated in a protein molecule in the process of formation. Thus, the DNA code is to be found in triplets—that is, three bases taken together code one amino acid.

The importance of the genetic code cannot be overstated. Let us assume the following sequence of bases in one of the strands of the DNA molecule: . . . CGT ATC GTA AGC . . . , and that the triplets in this sequence specify four amino acids, designated R, I, P, and E. In other words, the following code exists: CGT = R, ATC = I, GTA = P, and AGC = E. This section of the DNA molecule thus specifies RIPE, and the message to make RIPE is passed on by this particular sequence from the nucleus to the cytoplasm of the cell. The message continues to flow out in the living cell, and RIPE will be made, copy after copy.

But what if a chance mishap occurs in one of the triplets? Let us say that T in the second triplet is substituted for A, so that the triplet reads TTC instead of ATC, which would specify "A" instead of "I." The word would now be "RAPE" instead of "RIPE." This would be quite a difference, especially if the word is continually printed incorrectly throughout the novel. And just as a misprinted word can alter or destroy the meaning of a sentence, so does an altered protein in the body fail to express its intended purpose. Sometimes the error is not tragic, but more often than not, the person is debilitated by the misprint. As we have seen, in sickle-cell anemia, a single change in one of the bases of a triplet has fatal consequences.

Translation of the DNA Code

IN THE 1960's, it became evident that DNA did not directly form proteins but worked in a complex way through a secondary form of nucleic acid, ribonucleic acid, or RNA. As seen in FIGURE 11-5, a strand of DNA forms a one-stranded working copy of RNA. This RNA strand, which is responsible for carrying DNA's instructions out into the cell, is appropriately termed "messenger RNA." Messenger RNA is a negative print of DNA. The strand of RNA, however, has the nitrogenous base uracil (U) wherever thymine (T) would be present in

DNA. The four-letter alphabet or code accordingly applies to RNA rather than to DNA itself.

The genetic code, in its main elements, has been broken. Each three-letter of the messenger RNA is called a codon. Each of the 20 major amino acids, ranging from alanine to valine, has been shown to be specified by at least one codon. In fact, most amino acids have more than one codon. The amino acid serine, for example, has six codons, glycine has four, and lysine has two. Only methionine and tryptophan have one each. Because most amino acids are specified by more than one codon, the code is claimed to be "degenerate." However, this may be nature's device to insure that the code works.

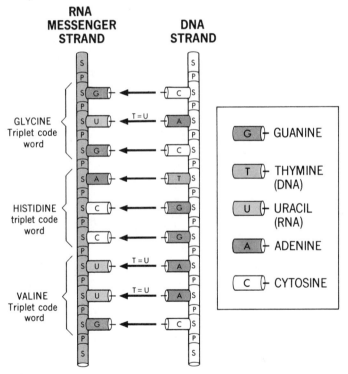

FIG. 11-5 THE LANGUAGE OF LIFE. The DNA molecule forms a single strand of "messenger" RNA which carries DNA's instructions out into the cell. The four bases of DNA (A, T, C, and G) are responsible for the three-letter code words in RNA. Each code word, or triplet, stands for one of the 20 amino acids that make up the variety of proteins in the body.

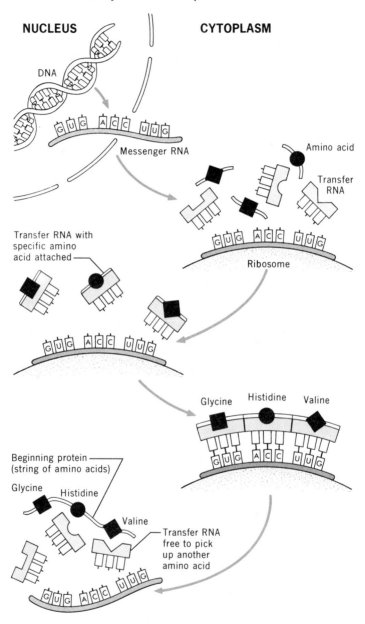

FIG. 11-6 THE MANUFACTURE OF PROTEIN. See text for explanations.

One of the most intriguing findings is that the code appears to be universal. The same triplet may code for the same amino acid in man as in the mouse. In an ingenious experiment, a strand of human DNA was fused with a strand of mouse DNA. The result, in the hybrid cell, was the production of some proteins common to man and mouse. The genetic code may be said to be the oldest of all languages.

The Ribosomal Assembly Line

SEVERAL EXPERIMENTS LED TO the conclusion that the sites of active protein synthesis are particles in the cytoplasm, called ribosomes. In the 1950's, M. B. Hoagland of Harvard Medical School discovered a molecular form of RNA smaller than that of messenger RNA. This smaller molecule was subsequently found to carry single, specific amino acids to the ribosomes. The molecule became known as transfer RNA.

The building of a specific protein then became clear (FIG. 11-6). Messenger RNA leaves the nucleus and threads itself through a ribosome, like a typewriter ribbon. As the ribosome "reads" a particular codon of messenger RNA, an appropriate type of transfer RNA is attracted to the ribosome. Each transfer RNA is designed so that it carries a specific amino acid on one end, and at the other end a sequence of three bases (called the anticodon) that fits only the corresponding codon in the messenger RNA. The transfer RNA molecule carrying glutamic acid, for example, recognizes the codon AAG in the messenger RNA molecule and brings its glutamic acid into position. Having served its purpose, the transfer RNA releases the glutamic acid, which becomes attached to the ribosome. As the messenger RNA continues to pass through the ribosome, the process is repeated with other molecules of transfer RNA, each adding its particular amino acids to those already attached in sequence to the ribosome. In this manner a series of linked amino acids is built up to form a protein.

The Abnormal Hemoglobins

THE BEST KNOWN of the abnormal hemoglobins is hemoglobin S, found in the blood cells of persons afflicted with sickle-cell

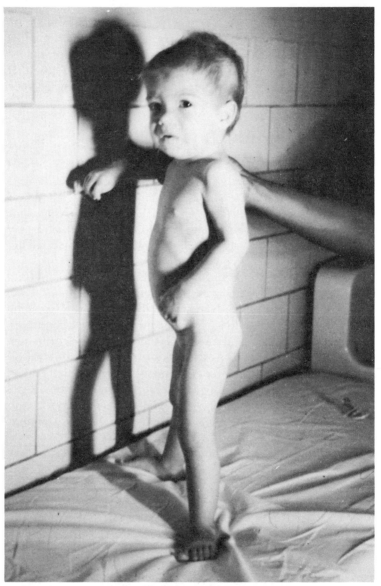

FIG. 11–7 PALE AND LISTLESS child suffering from thalassemia, or Cooley's ane-mia. This serious type of anemia occurs most commonly in persons of Mediter-ranean stock. (Courtesy of Dr. Norman Woody, Tulane University School of Medicine.)

anemia. This abnormality is caused by a mutation in one gene which codes a polypeptide chain 146 amino acid units in length. As we learned earlier, the mutation alters only one amino acid in the entire chain, changing a glutamic acid present in normal hemoglobin into another amino acid, valine. This change is the result of an alteration of a single base of the triplet of DNA which specifies the amino acid (specifically, the sixth amino acid of the 146 amino acid chain).

Another abnormal hemoglobin, hemoglobin C, has been isolated. The same glutamic acid unit that is replaced by valine in hemoglobin S is replaced by lysine in hemoglobin C. The mutant genes for hemoglobin C and S are allelic. That is to say, two independent mutations occurred in the same sequence of bases in DNA that make up a single gene. Here we may introduce our newer concept of the gene. A reasonable definition is that *the gene is that section of the DNA molecule involved in the determination of the amino acid sequence of a single polypeptide chain.* The "one gene—one enzyme" thesis thus gives way to the "one gene—one polypeptide" thesis.

The list of abnormal hemoglobins is growing rapidly; it now stretches to Q. The homozygous state for all of the variant hemoglobins leads to some form of blood disease. A serious, frequently fatal, type of anemia is thalassemia, or Cooley's anemia. It occurs most commonly in persons in the northern Mediterranean area, or in families of Mediterranean stock. The condition is recessively inherited. The severe homozygous condition is called thalassemia major; the heterozygous one is termed thalassemia minor. Heterozygous individuals may be mildly anemic.

The homozygote for thalassemia rarely survives into adult life. Homozygotes characteristically have massive spleens and bone deformities. The condition manifests itself early in life. The infant is pale and listless. A sunken nose and thick cranial bones give the impression that the child is suffering from mongolism (FIG. 11-7).

Thalassemia has become a problem of great magnitude in Italy. The number of thalassemic individuals has been estimated to surpass one million in this country alone. In several townships, one person in 10 is heterozygous and one child in every 100 has the severe homozygous condition. Since the heterozygote can be identified by blood tests, marriage advice has been widely advocated in Italy.

Life from the Laboratory

ONCE THE STRUCTURE OF DNA and RNA had been determined, researchers set to work to try to synthesize these nucleic acids. In 1955, Severo Ochoa succeeded in synthesizing a form of RNA that was chemically identical to RNA in the cell but which was not biologically active. The following year, Arthur Kornberg, then at Washington University at St. Louis, produced a molecule with all the physical and chemical properties of natural DNA, but not its biologic activity. Ochoa and Kornberg shared the 1959 Nobel Prize in medicine and physiology for these achievements.

In 1968, a major breakthrough was achieved by a team of researchers at Stanford University. Led by Nobel laureate Arthur Kornberg, the team produced an artificial copy of the DNA of a virus and demonstrated it to be as infectious as the original. The synthetic molecule replicates just as it would when a virus infects a cell. Kornberg essentially succeeded in copying a particular virus in a test tube. He was assisted by Mehran Goulian of the University of Chicago, formerly of the Stanford University Medical School, and Robert L. Sinsheimer of the California Institute of Technology.

The test-tube synthesis of a faithful copy of the original viral DNA is a remarkable feat. The hope is that medical researchers will soon be able to create modified forms of the virus and use them therapeutically. By infecting cells that have defective genes with man-made viruses that contain normal genes, the cells might be induced to produce the missing enzymes in genetic disorders. Kornberg's awesome accomplishment opens wide doors to new discoveries in combatting genetic disorders.

Epilogue

Genetic Engineering: Horror or Hope?

THROUGHOUT THE AGES, man has been eminently adept at modifying wild species of plants and animals to suit his needs and whims. He consciously determines which traits are to be incorporated or discarded in his domesticated stocks. Through continual "genetic engineering," man has perfected the sleek Arabian race horse, the toylike Shetland pony, the great Dane, and hordes of cultivated crops and ornamental plants.

Man also has yearned to improve his own kind. He would like to alter his genes according to his own design, thereby correcting or mitigating the hereditary defects that have plagued him. Less than two decades ago, the possibility of manipulating human genes represented the blue-sky ramblings of a handful of scientists. The outlook today is dramatically different. The spectacular achievements of recent years bring closer the day that many genetic defects—hemophilia, phenylketonuria, cystic fibrosis, sickle-cell anemia, and many others—can be corrected by rewriting the genetic code. The recent success of scientists in deciphering the genetic code, synthesizing biologically active DNA, and isolating pure genes has opened the door to a countless number of incredible experiments. Most of the basic information is now close at hand to artificially produce made-to-order genes. Once a functional synthetic gene is produced, it can be attached to a harmless virus which can serve to transmit the specific information of the gene. The harmless carrier virus can be introduced, for example, into a phenylketonuric child's liver, where the tailor-made gene can promote the production of the enzyme that has been errant in such patients.

Another fruitful avenue of approach is genetic surgery, which entails the repair or elimination, by chemicals or by radiation, of the base sequence of the defective piece of DNA in sufferers of serious genetic disorders. A major obstacle at present is the technical limitation of confining the action of the chemical or physical agent to only the undesired section of DNA. One tool that is being explored to slice through the DNA molecule at specific points is the laser, which emits incredibly fine beams of light.

One of the more startling possibilities is that of producing exact copies or replicas of any human being. This intriguing possibility stems from studies performed on the frog. Groups of adult frogs with identical genetical constitutions have been produced by the ingenious technique of implanting cells from one embryo individually into several unfertilized frog eggs. Apparently, then, a body cell, not merely the sperm and egg, contains all the genetic information needed to create a new individual. The procedures for the successful transplantation of a body cell into a mammalian egg have yet to be perfected. In the not too distant future, however, it seems likely that any man will be able to confer immortality upon himself simply by giving up a few of his body cells. An individual in one generation can prepare an additional copy of himself for another trial in the next generation.

The experimental tampering with human genes and traits has vast social and ethical implications. The potential for the misuse of knowledge is great. Nobel Prize winner Marshall W. Nirenberg cautions: "When man becomes capable of instructing his own cells, he must refrain from doing so until he has sufficient wisdom to use this knowledge for the benefit of mankind." Is man socially and morally prepared to cope with the newly emerging power of genetic engineering?

The current apprehension of medical scientists is reminiscent of the grave concern of an earlier group of scientists who opened Pandora's box in the 1940's with the terrifying mushroom-shaped atomic genie. But, just as there was no turning back then by the physical scientists, there seems to be no turning back now by the medical scientists. We may recall the perceptive words of Thomas Jefferson: "There is no truth on earth which I fear to be known."

Suggestions for Additional Readings

THERE ARE MANY exhaustive technical treatises on birth defects and hereditary diseases, but few have been written for the general reader. The books listed below dramatize the exciting progress in medical genetics for the nonprofessional reader, and can be read with much interest and enjoyment.

Tanner, James, Taylor, Gordon Rattray, and the editors of *Life. Growth.* New York: Time Inc., 1965.
   A simple, pictorial account of human development from conception to maturity.

Reed, Sheldon C. *Parenthood and Heredity.* 2nd Edition (Paperback). New York: John Wiley & Sons, Inc., 1964.
   Concise and interestingly presented book on counseling in human genetics. Inquires into the probability that parents with a family history of a given disorder will have children with the disorder in question.

Bergsma, Daniel, ed. *Conjoined Twins.* Birth Defects Original Article Series, Vol. III, No. 1, April 1967. New York: The National Foundation, 1967. (Available from The National Foundation—March of Dimes, 800 Second Avenue, New York 10017.)
   A lively, fascinating review of one of the most interesting anomalies in man—the conjoined twin.

Scheinfeld, Amram. *Your Heredity and Environment.* Philadelphia and New York: J. B. Lippincott Company, 1965.
   Delightful, profusely illustrated treatment of how heredity interacts with environment in every phase of a person's life.

Taylor, Gordon Rattray. *The Biological Time Bomb.* New York and Cleveland: New American Library, Inc., in association with The World Publishing Co., 1968.
   A sprightly, popular account of the impact on mankind of the new scientific discoveries and medical breakthroughs.

Dunn, L. C., and Dobzhansky, Th. *Heredity, Race, and Society*. 2nd Edition (Paperback). New York: New American Library, Inc., 1952.

An admirable little book on human differences, and the relative importance of nature and nurture.

Emery, Alan E. H. *Heredity, Disease, and Man: Genetics in Medicine*. Berkeley and Los Angeles: University of California Press, 1968.

A scholarly and readable treatment of the recent and challenging developments in genetics which are finding application in the practice of clinical medicine.

Hamerton, John L., ed. *Chromosomes in Medicine*. England: Wm. Heinemann (Medical Books) Ltd., 1962.

Valuable as a reference to the general reader who wishes to probe more deeply into congenital defects associated with mishaps in the chromosomes.

Knudson, Alfred G., Jr. *Genetics and Disease*. New York: McGraw-Hill, Inc., 1965.

Scholarly, vigorous treatment of human heredity and its relation to human disease. The presentation is at a high, but comprehensible, level.

Lerner, I. Michael. *Heredity, Evolution, and Society*. San Francisco: W. H. Freeman and Company, 1968.

An authoritative, modern consideration of the social and political ramifications of the biological laws governing heredity and evolution. The presentation is broad and deep, but intelligible to the average reader.

Index

(Page numbers in bold face refer to illustrations)